Living the Thin Life

A Dieting and Weight Loss
Guide with Weight Loss Tips
& Weight Maintenance
Strategies for Life

Elle Marie

For Dad, who always inspired me by his example and his love of books

This book is not intended as a substitute for medical advice from physicians. The reader should consult a physician in matters relating to his or her health, including any significant change in dietary practices.

Contents

Acknowledgements

I would like to thank Victoria Monti, my daughter, for her enthusiasm, patience, and tough but gentle editing. I want to thank Stephen Monti, my son, for contributing his original artwork. I also would like to thank Dannette McKellar for her great suggestions and writing tips. Thanks to all my wonderful friends and family who provided their stories and secrets.

Special thanks go to Doug for all of his support and understanding.

Introduction

I'm not a doctor or a nutritionist. I don't work for a weight-loss clinic or a fitness company. I'm not trying to sell you anything. I am just an ordinary, middle-aged woman who has managed to lose the weight I needed to lose and then keep it off. I am living the thin life, and it's a great life! I don't feel self-conscious like I used to when I was carrying around those extra pounds. Now I have the confidence to enjoy life as I've always wanted to.

Over the years, I've read just about every diet book and visited every diet website I could find, looking for ways to successfully maintain my ideal weight with a minimum of sacrifice. I've experimented with lots of ideas, and discovered that some but not all of them work for me. I've learned how to adapt all that information and advice to fit my own individual lifestyle and personality. And I think that's the secret—to be willing to try out new recipes, exercises, and motivation strategies. Then I discard the ones that don't work for me and add the ones that do work to my regular routine. Over time, these strategies become habits. I don't feel like I'm on a diet, but rather that I have a lifetime eating plan.

To lose weight, you must take in fewer calories than you expend in energy. To maintain a level weight, the energy input (food) must remain equal to the energy output (exercise). Sounds simple, right? Somehow it becomes complicated when you compare different approaches that contradict each other or that require weighing, measuring, and counting. The trick to making it easy is finding ways of getting the right amount of exercise and eating a healthy diet that will be effective for you. If the techniques you try require too much effort or don't suit your personality and lifestyle, you will lose heart and give up on them.

In this book, I will help you identify your own unique motivators to keep you on track, develop a food plan that fits into your lifestyle, and build an exercise program that you can stick with. You will end up with a personalized system that will allow you to stay at a healthy weight for the rest of your life. I have researched tips from many diet experts and looked at the many rules they provide. While I agree that a lot of the tips make sense and will work for most people, I also believe that every person is different and you sometimes need to break the rules and make up your own rules.

My story is not dramatic. As I said, I'm an ordinary American woman, an office worker from the baby boomer generation. For most of my life, I was at a normal weight. When I was in my twenties, my two children were born. I had no trouble staying slim with two very active kids and a full-time job. As the years went by, I found myself picking up one or two extra pounds each year. Although it didn't seem like much, those pounds were adding up. I was cooking family-style meals high in carbohydrates and fat. We ate lots of pasta, casseroles, bread, and desserts.

I guess my metabolism started slowing down as I became more sedentary. After returning from a one-week Caribbean cruise to celebrate my wedding anniversary, I stepped on the scale and realized I was 20 pounds over my ideal weight! That was when I finally decided to take action and make some changes in my life. My clothes were tight and unflattering, my energy level was low, and I just didn't feel good about myself. I set a goal to lose those extra 20 pounds and keep them off forever.

By this time my son and daughter were grown up and independent and my husband was very supportive. I had more free time to focus on myself and come up with a lifelong plan I could stick to. This was my opportunity to take control of my eating and exercise habits.

I started out with a low-carbohydrate diet, which I was able to stick with for eight weeks. After losing about eight pounds, I switched to a low-calorie plan and continued losing, although at a slower pace. I started taking aerobics classes at a local gym, then joined a women-only fitness center that combined strength training with aerobics. I reached my goal weight and loved it! My clothes now looked great on me and I got lots of compliments. I felt energized!

The next challenge was figuring out how to maintain my ideal weight for the rest of my life (*without* feeling like I was always on a diet).

Don't think I'm one of those naturally thin people who can eat whatever they want and never gain an ounce. I have to work at it like everyone else. I have always enjoyed food and love to snack. I had to find ways to satisfy my sweet tooth without putting the pounds back on. I never liked to work out, so I had to find ways to work exercise into my daily routine and keep myself motivated.

In this book, I'll share the tips and tricks that have worked for me. I've included stories from friends and family members who succeeded in losing weight and keeping it off. I'll show you how to create your own personal system tailored to your likes and dislikes. I will include some shortcuts that will make sticking to your plan easier. I'll also provide fun quizzes to test your knowledge. In Appendix C, I offer many easy, delicious recipes.

My husband asked me not to use his real name in this book, so I'll just call him "Elvis" (he's the king, or at least he likes to think so). Elvis and I have had many discussions about proper eating and exercise habits. His ideas are usually very different from mine. I'll try to be objective and tell you about his suggestions, too. You be the judge, but keep in mind he is about 30 pounds overweight while I have maintained my ideal weight for over ten years.

For example, Elvis has three cookies for breakfast each morning. He explains, "You're not supposed to take a vitamin on an empty stomach." While it's true you should take vitamins with meals, you don't need 450 extra calories, with the main ingredient being sugar.

Elvis also has the attitude that some diet foods are not "real". Most people know that skim milk is regular cow's milk that has had most of the cream skimmed off. It has the same nutrients as whole milk, but with less fat. Having spent some time on a farm as a child, I've actually seen the skimming process. But Elvis feels that skim milk isn't real. Maybe he thinks there's some kind of dairy animal called a skim.

Throughout the book, I'll also try to provide some examples of what *not* to do. You may see Elvis's name come up in these examples.

I'm now in my fifties and I feel better than I ever have. I have lots of energy plus Elvis tells me I look better now than I did when we got married. So don't be discouraged. It *is* possible to keep the weight off and live the thin life!

Part One

Pep Talk

Chapter 1

Let's Get Motivated

This is my key message: Discover what motivates *you* and what works for *you*. We are all unique individuals. We don't look alike or think alike, so why should we expect the same eating or exercise program to work for everyone? In fact, research has shown that women differ from one another more than men do[1]. These differences make it important to develop your own system and not expect a "one-size-fits-all" program to work for you. Pick and choose from all the suggestions and advice presented here to come up with your own personalized plan. Improvise by adjusting, combining, or adding suggestions.

Over the years I've realized you can develop a system that suits you through experimentation and learning from your experiences. It's an ongoing process that you will continue to fine-tune over time. There are new products continually being developed—exercise equipment and programs, sugar and fat substitutes, new menu items at restaurants—so you can add variety to your routine and avoid monotony. That keeps it fun!

The first step in developing your custom plan is to

discover your own personal motivators. What truly makes you want to do whatever it takes to stay healthy and fit? When you're tempted to overeat or skip a workout, what thoughts will keep you on track by reminding you of why you want to stay in good shape? Here are some possibilities to consider:

A desire to be healthy. This is a great motivator for most people. Maintaining a healthy weight can help reduce your risk of developing certain health conditions such as:

- High blood pressure
- Type 2 diabetes
- Heart disease and stroke
- High blood fats such as cholesterol and triglycerides
- Arthritis
- Cancer
- Gallstones
- Fatty liver disease

Being overweight can also contribute to sleep apnea, which can strain your heart and make you feel fatigued throughout the day. Extra fatty tissue in the throat can cause snoring which may disrupt your sleep.

Overweight people are more affected by air pollution than people of normal weight, according to a 2007 study[2]. Pollution causes temporary drops in lung function that decrease lung efficiency. Normal and underweight people in the study didn't have this reaction.

Being fit is a great feeling. You will wake up each morning looking forward to a new day. While there are health factors we can't control, taking charge of your health is empowering. You will feel confident about yourself, knowing you are taking the best care of your body you can.

If that's not enough to keep you motivated, here are

more benefits of being thin and fit that have been demonstrated in various research studies:

- Fit people over age 40 have a 50% lower risk of stroke.[3]
- Physically active older adults live longer.[4]
- Older adults who maintain their strength have fewer balance problems.[5]

When you're having trouble sticking to your exercise and eating plan, think about all the health benefits of being fit.

Looking good! We all want to look our best. Having a trim and toned body will help to make your clothes look great on you. You'll love to catch sight of your reflection in a mirror or store window. Knowing you are attractive is a great confidence-builder.

If you are overweight, you may feel self-conscious about the impression you make on others. Being at your ideal weight can remove this worry and allow you to be yourself so people can focus on your other qualities. Appearance can be a great motivator.

We all need to be realistic about our body image. You don't have to be a size two or look like an ultra thin model or actress to look good. Understand what weight *you* look your best in, taking into consideration your own bone structure, body shape, and genetics. Then you can just relax and accept yourself.

Deferred gratification. Say no now, knowing you can say yes later. This strategy really works for me. If I'm having dinner out or at a friend's house, I can pass on dessert, because I know I have a tasty healthy treat waiting for me at home. When you have to wait for something, getting it is a greater pleasure. Remember the anticipation you felt as a child in the weeks leading up to Christmas or your birthday? If we received presents every day, they would lose their value to us. That same attitude applies to food. Food tastes better when you're hungrier. Let yourself take the time to feel a little hunger, and the eventual reward will be sweeter.

I like to keep great-tasting low-calorie desserts around the house, such as sugar-free, fat-free pudding. With something to look forward to throughout the day, it is easier to turn down other foods. One of my favorite ways to relax in the evening is to work a crossword puzzle or read a book while enjoying a sweet snack. If I have my dessert or treat earlier, I no longer have my special indulgence to look forward to. A treat tastes much better when you have waited for it.

Really **deferred gratification**. Once a week, Elvis and I go out to dinner. We enjoy relaxing at a nice restaurant on a Friday night after working all week. It's a special treat since we eat at home the other six nights of the week. When we eat out, we order what we like. I may skip the bread, but I don't order "diet" food. When I'm tempted to splurge during the week, I remind myself that I'll be having a nice meal on Friday and I can wait.

Try this technique yourself by planning some future reward you can look forward to. It's much easier to pass up your favorite foods when you know you will get to enjoy them later. Surely you can wait just a few more days! That special meal will taste better, and you will have saved extra calories by waiting.

Getting compliments. I enjoy it when Elvis tells me I'm the prettiest girl at the party or I look better now than I did in my thirties. It's fun to get compliments from friends and family too. You can stay motivated in the face of temptation by remembering that warm feeling of appreciation.

It's fun for me to be out with my grown daughter and be mistaken for sisters. Many people I meet don't believe I have children in their late twenties. I've been accused of being a "child bride"!

> "A recent large study at the University of Maryland has shown that thin women have fewer hot flashes than heavy women.[6]"

Feeling in control. Maintaining your desired weight gives you a great feeling of control. You are making the choices that determine how you look and feel. You understand your individual likes and dislikes and work them into your overall plan. You're not at the mercy of hunger pangs because you have figured out how to eat sensibly. You don't dread a workout because you have decided to make regular exercise a part of your life.

Not getting out of breath. One of the great things about being in good physical condition is your increase in endurance. Over time, you will strengthen not only your muscles, but your lungs as well. You'll be able to walk or climb stairs more easily. When you're tempted to skip a workout, remind yourself how much you appreciate being able to do more without getting winded or fatigued. It will all be worth it.

Shopping for new clothes. When you're slim, you can wear clothes in styles you choose, not what happens to fit from a limited selection. You can wear clothes in all your favorite colors instead of sticking with dark solid colors. You can wear belts to show off your waistline. Clothes look best on people with trim, toned bodies. Fashionable clothing is designed to fit and flatter slim people.

Looking forward to holidays and special occasions. Some people are motivated by a special occasion for which they want to look their best. For example, if you have a high school reunion coming up in six months, you can use the desire to impress your old friends as a motivator to keep you on your eating and exercise plan for the next six months. After you have enjoyed your special event, pick the next one coming up on the horizon, such as the Christmas holidays or a summer vacation. Motivating yourself in six-month increments can be very effective and can help build lifetime habits.

Knowing you're in good shape will help you look forward to special occasions rather than dreading them. Also keep in mind that at special events (especially weddings and holidays) people usually take lots of pictures and save those pictures for life, so that's extra incentive to look good in them.

Being there for your family. Dennis C., a relative of mine, maintains his motivation by thinking about all the future years he wants to enjoy with his children and someday (hopefully) grandchildren. He knows that being heavy can shorten your lifespan and reduce the quality of life in the years you do have. He wants to be an active, important part of the lives of the people he cares about for as long as possible.

Your family and friends can be a strong motivating factor for you. Besides looking to the future, you will get more enjoyment out of the time you spend with them today when you are strong and healthy. It's a wonderful feeling to make them proud of you. When I told my son I was planning to write this book, he said, "Be sure to put lots of pictures of yourself in it." That comment sure gave *me* motivation!

Having strength for everyday tasks. Simple tasks like

carrying bags of groceries or doing laundry are much easier when you're in good physical condition. It's great to be able to handle going up stairs without dreading it as an ordeal to get through. If you're out of shape, simple things like opening a heavy door at a department store, taking out the trash, or even pushing a grocery cart can become challenging.

On the other hand, being in good shape improves your endurance, so you are able to go on walking tours on a vacation or even hiking in national parks. You don't want to be one of those people who straggles behind and slows everyone else down, do you? Think of all the things you do that are easy when you're physically fit, but difficult when you're not—such as hoisting your carry-on bag into the overhead compartment on an airplane, bending over to pick up something you've dropped, or getting something off a high shelf. Life is just easier all around when you're physically fit.

Boosting your energy level. When you're healthy and fit, you'll naturally feel more energetic vs. feeling sluggish. And who wants to feel like a slug? That doesn't sound very appealing to me.

Have you ever been stuck behind one of those slow-moving people you just can't get around at the shopping mall or grocery store? It can be frustrating when you want to move quickly. Which of these people do you want to be: the slow-moving obstacle or the determined, quick-moving go-getter?

I've talked with women who started exercising after years of inactivity. One friend told me that before she started working out regularly, she would dread forgetting something and then having to walk extra steps to go back and get it. She didn't realize how little energy she had until she lost weight and gained strength. Now it's no problem for her to take extra steps, and in fact she will sometimes intentionally go out of her way to get more steps in.

Having a never-ending wardrobe. You can save money on clothes because you'll only need one size. When your weight fluctuates a lot from going on and off diets, you may accumulate lots of clothes in different sizes. Or if you have been steadily gaining weight over the years, you may have been gradually buying larger sizes and now find yourself with a closet full of clothes that don't fit. When you are able to maintain the same size, every item in your closet is wearable. You'll never have to throw anything out.

I've been at a stable weight for many years and it's almost embarrassing how old some of my favorite clothes are. As long as they fit well, why not go ahead and keep wearing them? I still get compliments on outfits that are more than 20 years old! It's helpful to buy good quality, classic-styled clothing, knowing it will last the years. Of course, some of the clothes that still fit me I wouldn't be caught dead in! I just hang on to them hoping that they'll be back in style someday.

Improved self-esteem. If you are in good shape, you can avoid feelings of embarrassment. On the other hand, when you know you're not at your best you may not look forward to meeting new people because you're worried about the impression you may be making. Instead of being open to new situations and opportunities, you may be too focused on your self-perceived flaws to appreciate other people and experiences.

Feeling good about yourself will give you the self-confidence and freedom to enjoy what life has to offer. The energy you might have spent worrying about your appearance can now be used for more productive purposes.

Competition—being a winner. This suggestion might not work for everyone, but there are some people who thrive on competition. A certain relative of mine motivates himself to lose weight by making a bet with someone, usually his brother. He puts up a significant amount of money and then either sets a deadline for when he needs to lose a certain amount of weight, or just races the other person to see who can lose a certain amount first. He is so competitive that he usually loses weight out of sheer determination to win the bet.

You may want to try this motivator with a reward other than cash. How about competing with a friend to see who can complete more workouts in a certain period of time, and then treating the winner to a day at the spa? How about creating a trophy to award to the friend who loses the most weight? Or maybe just the satisfaction of winning is enough for you.

Flexibility and youthfulness. The most important factor in projecting a youthful appearance is having flexibility in your movements. Many older people move very slowly and stiffly. Of course, we all will age eventually and if you have stiffness due to injuries or arthritis there may not be much you can do. However, for most of us, stiffness can be delayed by participating in some sort of regular exercise. A person who walks briskly and moves easily will appear much more youthful.

Investing in yourself. Maybe you're the type of person who hates to waste money. Try signing up for a weight loss class, exercise program, or dance lessons. Once you've committed your cash, you'll be motivated to stick with it, if only to feel like you're getting your money's worth.

Enjoying more space. One of the great things about

being thin is simply not taking up so much physical space. With a smaller body, you have more room to breathe. When you're flying in coach class on an airplane or taking a subway, you can easily fit into your seat. I always feel sorry for the heavy-set people I see trying to squeeze into those tiny spaces. You also have more room in movie theaters, dressing rooms, and even bathroom stalls. Keep reminding yourself how comfortable it is to have your personal space and you'll be sure to maintain your motivation.

Taking up more space can also have some unexpected negative consequences. Two heavy relatives of mine were actually kicked off an amusement park ride once because they were too large. It was extremely embarrassing to them.

You can decide to never let this happen to you. When you're tempted to eat unwisely or skip a workout, remind yourself of this.

> "Fat may damage brain cells—a French study of 2,000 middle-aged people found that the higher the Body Mass Index, the lower the memory test scores.[7]"

Emulating someone. Maybe I'm a little shallow, but having a role model to emulate is motivating for me. I may pass someone on the street or see an actress in a movie who looks great, and I think to myself, "That's what I want to look like!"

An alternative is to use yourself as your role model. Keep a picture of yourself when you were in peak shape, and use it to remind yourself of how good you can be. This picture lets you become your own role model and creates motivation and enthusiasm for maintaining your weight.

Not **emulating someone**. For some people, having a negative role model is motivating. Remind yourself of what you *don't* want to look like. With the growing number of overweight and obese Americans, you can easily find someone who is not at her optimum weight and physical condition. You can stay motivated in order to avoid becoming that person. Some people will even display pictures of obese people on their refrigerators to motivate themselves to forgo an impulsive snack.

Maintaining self-discipline or willpower. This is the absolute last item on my list, because it's the one that rarely works, at least not for the long-term. I'll include it anyway because it's possible it will work for you. If you can make a commitment to exercise and to eat healthy because you know it's a good decision and the right thing to do for yourself, that commitment may give you the strength to stick to it.

Your homework assignment

You are about to create the first part of your personal plan for life. Use the personal plan worksheet in Appendix A.

1. Select at least three ideas from the list above which apply to you. Really think about what's important to you personally that makes you want to be slim and trim. Write these items down in Section 1 of your plan. You'll need this motivation list later when you're fighting temptation to remind yourself why you want to stick to your plan.

2. Add your own ideas by thinking about times when you were successful in sticking to a diet or exercise routine. Don't worry about your ideas appearing to be silly to someone else. Remember, this is *your* list of what motivates you.

Chapter 2

No Excuses!

Okay, so now you've found your own personal motivators and have made up your mind that you are going to maintain (or improve) your weight and fitness level. You believe you're ready to develop your own custom maintenance plan and you know it will be something you can live with.

However, even though you're highly motivated, you may have some negative thoughts that can sabotage your plan. These may be hidden beliefs you're not even consciously aware of but which can hold you back and keep you from fully committing to a healthy lifestyle.

Let's bring these excuses out into the open and examine them. In the light of day, you can recognize what your obstacles may be and challenge yourself to overcome them. It's possible that by simply becoming aware of them you will understand how to counter their influence over your behavior.

Here are some common excuses I've heard on why people don't stick to an eating or fitness plan:

I'm naturally fat—it's in my genes. Some people may

have an inherited tendency to be overweight, but this doesn't mean it's hopeless for you. I know many families (including my own) that include heavy people as well as thin people. We may have all come from the same gene pool, but we've made different lifestyle choices that influence our health and weight.

If you are one of those unlucky people who have to work harder than most to maintain a healthy weight, you might as well learn to accept it. Over time, as you build wholesome habits, a healthy lifestyle will become more natural to you and will seem like less effort. Don't just give up and blame Mom and Dad for your situation.

At the gym where I work out, I met a woman who recently lost a significant amount of weight and looks great. She admitted that she had been overweight since she was five years old. Yet she was able to overcome a lifetime of being heavy through proper diet and exercise. She said once she learned how to create a healthy eating plan, she had no trouble sticking to it. Eating right is now a habit for her.

Eating in an unhealthy way can be a habit some people pick up as kids. Another woman I know started overeating as a child when her mother died and her father wasn't able to cook for the family. She developed the habit of only eating fast food.

> "An obese person faces a 50% greater risk of illness than a person of normal weight. If the obese person is physically fit, the risk drops to 30%.[1]"

However, eating healthy can become a habit too; it just takes some time to form. Once you get past the first 30 days or so, it will become easier.

I'll never lose the weight I gained when I was pregnant. Some women may believe this common excuse, but I'm sure we all know people who have given birth to several children and have somehow managed to return to their pre-pregnancy weight. Most of your pregnancy weight gain should be in support of the baby you are nurturing and should drop off easily after the baby is born. If that wasn't the case for you, then you've probably added a general gain in fat by consuming more calories during your pregnancy than the baby needed. This is the same kind of weight gain that will result from any type of overeating, and the pregnancy excuse is simply a way of trying to disavow responsibility. But the good news is that since it is ordinary weight gain, the same techniques for losing weight in general also apply to pregnancy weight gain. There is no special secret to losing this type of weight versus any other type.

It does take time to lose the weight, but the more slowly you lose the weight, the more likely it is to stay off permanently. I gained about 25 pounds during each of my pregnancies. After each baby was born, I couldn't fit into my normal clothes and actually had to wear my husband's jeans for a while. After about three months, I was almost back to normal. I could wear my own clothes, although I admit they were still a little snug around the waist. Finally, after six months, I was back at my pre-pregnancy weight. I was able to achieve this by eating carefully and getting lots of exercise, mainly from chasing my kids!

I'm getting older and as people age, they naturally gain weight. There is some truth to this argument. In fact, you don't want to be *too* thin as you get older, as that can put you at risk for a slower recovery from normal illnesses. Most of us, however, don't have the problem of being too thin.

The weight that was optimum for you at age 18, 25, or 35, is still close to your optimum weight at age 50 and older. The reason we gain weight as we get older is that we continue the same eating habits we had in our twenties, while actually requiring fewer calories. The average 50-year-old woman needs around 300-500 fewer calories per day than she did when she was 25 to maintain the same body weight[2].

I'll give you an example of a pair of identical twins in their seventies. Let's call them "Moan" and "Joan". For most of their lives, they have been equal in weight and fitness. At one point, however, Moan started making some different lifestyle choices than Joan. Moan eats many high carbohydrate and high fat foods and rarely exercises. Her favorite activities are talking on the telephone and watching television. Joan, on the other hand, goes to regular exercise classes, takes long, frequent walks, and is careful about what she eats. She has much more stamina than the first twin, has lower blood pressure, and has a more healthy weight. Moan tells people she's just getting old, while Joan doesn't even think about aging. This contrast is clear evidence that you don't have to lose your fitness level as you get older.

I *need* my regular soda and I hate diet soda. This is an example of not being willing to try some new things. Sure, maybe you really love your regular soda and you've gotten in the habit of drinking six cans a day, but it really is possible to change. You know you don't really *need* soda. You just enjoy it or maybe it's your comfort food.

Why not start out by replacing one serving of soda per day with water or a diet soda? Do this for one week, then reduce your regular soda intake a little more the next week. You may find diet soda isn't really so bad once you get used to the taste of it. Or you may grow to love the fresh, healthy feeling you get when you're well hydrated from drinking enough water. There are also other low-calorie drink choices, such as sugar-free cranberry juice or lemonade. Be open to new tastes and you may be surprised to find out that you can live without soda after all.

If that doesn't work for you, then you can decide to go ahead and allow yourself that one treat that means so much to you. However, you'll have to find another way of compensating for all those calories you're consuming. So, if you must have the soda, you need to either give something else up, or maybe drink one glass of water for every soda you have, or use the soda as a reward after exercise. Be creative!

My metabolism is slower than most people. Well, maybe it is, and maybe it isn't. You do have some control over your metabolism. Eating right and exercising regularly will have a beneficial effect on your metabolism.

> "Your metabolism naturally slows down by about 2% to 5% per decade after age 40[3]."

If your metabolism does happen to be slower than most people, you need to learn about the things you can do to improve the situation. Don't just give up and accept being at a non-healthy weight.

Some ways to increase your metabolic rate are:

- Eat protein, especially first thing in the morning. I like to have a hardboiled egg for breakfast each day. You may prefer a small amount of breakfast meat (but watch out for excessive amounts of fat).

Elle Marie

- Exercise for at least 30 minutes three times each week. Don't be afraid to do more than the minimum. Exercising five times a week or for an hour each time is even better.
- Don't eat a lot of food at one sitting. Spread your calories out across the day.
- Don't allow long periods of time between meals or snacks. Your body may start to move into "starvation mode" to conserve energy by slowing down your metabolic rate.

Following a diet and exercise plan is too complicated. It doesn't have to be complicated! There are many simple ways to construct a meal plan and exercise program that are effective for you. In Chapter 5, I'll offer a quiz you can take to determine your eating style. In Chapter 6, I'll provide tips you can use to develop healthy eating habits which fit your style and personality. Not every diet plan involves complex calculations or balancing grams of fat against grams of protein or carbohydrates. For many people, simple guidelines are the most effective and easiest to incorporate into their existing routines.

The same concept applies to exercise. While some exercises require fancy (and expensive!) equipment or membership at a gym, there are many things you can do at home or as part of your regular daily activities. Stay tuned for Chapter 9, where I'll give you lots of ways to build physical activity into your lifestyle.

I just don't like diet food. Maybe you haven't tried any recently. You may be amazed at the low calorie and low fat foods available today. New products are coming out all the time, with tremendous improvements in quality and taste. Diet ice cream is creamier, low calorie pudding is sweeter, and diet soda tastes almost just like the original. Sugar and fat substitutes allow you to eat great-tasting food without packing on the pounds, yet provide a similar level of satisfaction as the original foods.

There are other ways to maintain your weight without eating "diet" food all the time. One way is to eat smaller portion sizes of your favorite foods. Another is to make up for extra calories consumed by exercising. In Chapters 6 and 7, I'll provide many ideas you can try for designing an eating plan that works for you.

I don't have time to worry about my weight. Many people have very busy lives and so they choose to do things the easy or quick way. They may eat at fast food restaurants rather than preparing home-cooked meals. They may have tight schedules filled with work, children's activities, and other responsibilities that don't seem to leave any time for exercise. Does this sound like you?

If it does, don't give up. Developing a customized eating plan will definitely require some planning and some experimentation. You may have to measure portion sizes until you learn to make accurate estimates. You may have to look up calorie counts until you have them memorized for your favorite foods. You may need to keep a food diary until you have developed a good feel for what foods and quantities you are consuming each day. Over time, though, you should be able to discard the time-consuming research and tracking.

Other techniques, such as eliminating whole categories of food from your diet, don't require measuring or logging. These may work better for you. Another option is to incorporate one small change at a time to minimize the planning and preparation for your new eating plan. After that change has been worked into your routine, try adding another one.

It may take some time and effort at first to find

effective strategies, but once you have figured out what works for you, make them part of your life. It's definitely worth it!

It's okay if I'm a little overweight—everyone else is. Americans have a high obesity rate which seems to be getting worse all the time, but that doesn't mean it's healthy. Do you remember your mother asking you, "If everyone else jumped off a cliff, would you do it, too?" You don't have to be like everybody else when it comes to bad habits. Raise the bar on your standards for yourself!

Exercise is boring. There are many ways to make exercise more interesting. One suggestion is to vary your routine so you're not doing the same old exercises day after day, week after week. In Chapter 8, you'll read about many options for exercising. Try different activities to break up the repetition.

I personally think the best way to keep exercise from being boring is to simply add physical exertion into your lifestyle. Maybe you don't need to set aside certain times to exercise if you start parking further away from the store, taking the stairs instead of the elevator, or walking over to talk to a co-worker face to face rather than sitting at your desk sending an email.

You can also make a boring exercise fun by doing it to music. A woman I met at my gym told me she loves the treadmill. She can keep jogging on her treadmill until she loses all track of the time just by listening to her favorite songs on her iPod. Even Elvis will use his treadmill as long as he can watch the evening news on television while he's exercising. It's a simple way to time your exercise, too. When your half-hour TV show is over, you know you've put in 30 minutes of exercise.

I don't want to give up my favorite foods, even though they're unhealthy. You may need to make some tough choices here. Rather than totally give up a food you love, you can cut down on the quantity you consume. For example, I love dark chocolate. I could eat it all day if I allowed myself. Instead of completely giving it up, I only eat one or two Dove chocolates at a time, and I don't eat them every day. When I do eat one, I savor it and make it last as long as I can so it's really worth the fat and calories.

You could also try a reduced-calorie or low-fat version of your favorite food. I never thought I would get Elvis to eat lite ice cream. He used to always insist on the creamiest, fattiest, most sugary, highest calorie version he could find whenever we bought ice cream at the grocery store. One day, I somehow managed to get him to try a slow-churned, low-fat brand. Surprisingly enough, he loved it! Now my next challenge is to get him to eat a reasonable serving size.

Another suggestion, which probably won't be very popular, is to eliminate the "bad" foods from your diet altogether and keep yourself motivated by reminding yourself of all the good reasons you want to be a healthy weight. I never said this would be easy, but I can guarantee you the pleasure you will get from being slim and feeling good will outweigh any feelings of being deprived.

Your homework assignment

1. Choose which of the excuses above may apply to you.
2. Think of any other excuses you may have for avoiding a commitment to a weight maintenance plan. Enter them into Section 2 of your custom plan.

Chapter 3

When Temptation Hits

No matter how determined you are to stick to your plan, temptations will arise to try to lead you astray. Maybe your spouse is having a big bowl of ice cream in front of you. Elvis loves to do this to me. Maybe a friend invites you to a party, potluck dinner, or a night on the town. A commercial on television for your favorite food can tempt you, and so can a delicious aroma coming from a bakery. There are many situations that will test your resolve and make it difficult for you to make healthy choices.

Temptations are uniquely personal. What is absolutely irresistible to you may not be tempting at all to your best friend, but on the other hand, you may be able to easily pass up something that she feels helpless to ignore. Understanding your own weaknesses is the first step in developing personalized methods for dealing with them.

So what can you do when temptation hits? How can you resist? How can you develop effective defenses to protect yourself and help you stick to your lifetime plan for being healthy and fit?

The answer is to plan ahead. Determine which strategies are effective for you, and then make use of them whenever you are faced with the urge to overeat or underexercise.

Here are some ideas that I have found helpful in resisting temptations:

Stay out of temptation's way. Avoiding the temptation in the first place is much easier than figuring out how to resist it. Try not to keep high-calorie foods in the house that may tempt you to overeat. If they are there right in front of you, they can be nearly impossible to resist.

Perhaps you like to have candy sitting out in bowls around your house or office for guests. There's a good chance you may end up eating at least some of it yourself. One solution that still allows you to be hospitable is to set out foods that are not especially tempting to you. For example, while I love dark chocolate, I have no problem at all turning down milk chocolate. If I provide candy bowls with milk chocolate candy bars, I can easily resist eating them myself, but my guests can still enjoy a treat when they visit. That is, if there's any left after Elvis gets to it.

Try not to even buy junk food. If it's there, you may end up eating it, but if it's not there, you probably won't want to run all the way to the store to get it. Eventually your craving will pass.

If you can't remove the tempting foods completely because of other household members or visitors, at least make it inconvenient for you to get to them. Maybe you can store the cookies on a high shelf in your pantry or put the ice cream in the back of your freezer behind other items. You may just forget they are even there.

I also recommend keeping lots of diet-friendly snacks on hand so you have something to satisfy you when a craving hits. How about fresh fruit, low fat ice cream, or sugar-free pudding? Just remember to watch the portion sizes!

Don't go out to eat. This may not be totally realistic, but you can at least try to limit the number of times you eat out each week. You will have much more control over your eating when you're at home, surrounded by the healthy foods you have chosen.

If you don't want to be completely unsociable, go ahead and go out occasionally, but try to choose restaurants that offer lower calorie options or "light" menu items. Skip the sauces and go for plain grilled fish or meat. You might want to stick to soup and salad or have an appetizer for your main dish instead of a fattening entrée.

Fast food is cheap, filling, and readily available when you're in a hurry so it can be very tempting. If you must eat fast food, try to improve the quality of your nutrition when on the run. One way is to order smaller portions. You'll save over 100 calories if you get a small order of fries instead of the supersized order, and it will probably still satisfy your craving. You can order a small sandwich or even a kid's meal for a smaller serving.

If you order a side salad, you'll be less likely to fill up on the higher calorie items. The salad will also provide some fiber and vitamins to balance an otherwise unhealthy meal. Instead of a hamburger place, try going to one of the deli-style fast food chains where you can order a sub or sandwich on whole wheat bread or a wrap, which will save you calories and fat grams compared to fried food.

Keep in mind chicken isn't always a healthy choice. Many fried, breaded chicken sandwiches on white bread are actually higher in fat and calories than a hamburger. Grilled chicken is a better option.

Avoid all-you-can-eat buffets. This may be the worst possible situation you can be in when it comes to temptation. There's bound to be something on the buffet that is tempting to everyone.

At events where food is served buffet style, a good strategy is to first survey the entire selection of food. Scope out all the choices and plan what you will put on your plate before you even get in line. If you know fruit is among the dessert offerings, for example, you can pass by the other desserts.

At a buffet, only take food you are likely to enjoy without straying too far from your regular foods. Don't waste calories on food you don't really love. You can get rid of some of the calories by scraping off sauces (I always scrape off cheesy sauces that don't appeal to me anyway), removing skin from chicken and turkey, and trying to blot up any excess oil or grease with a napkin.

If you have control over what is being served, try to limit the selection of food choices. When you are faced with a variety of different foods, you may be tempted to try a little (or a lot) of everything. For Thanksgiving, don't serve pumpkin, cherry, *and* chocolate cream pies. Just pick one type of pie and then you can allow yourself one piece.

Wear clothes that fit you well. This is especially important when going out to parties or get-togethers with friends and family. Don't wear drawstring pants, skirts with elastic waistbands, or anything that's loose around the middle. That will just make it easier for you to eat too much before you know it.

On the other hand, if you're wearing clothes that already fit snugly and then you start to overdo it, the clothing will begin to feel tight and uncomfortable, reminding you that you really don't want to overeat.

Or you could be like Elvis. One of his most adorable

sit in his recliner after a big meal and undo
ı on his pants. Maybe I should get him a

Really enjoy your treats. If you have a craving for a treat such as chocolate, go ahead and have some. But make sure you savor the experience. Take the time to purchase some high-end gourmet chocolate and then sit down and eat it slowly. You may have to go out and get it if you don't have it around the house, making it even more of a treat.

Occasionally having a small amount of your favorite food will help you stay on track with your eating plan. Remember to eat it leisurely and enjoy each bite. Make it last so you'll feel it was worthwhile. If you just scarf it down, you won't feel as satisfied. There's nothing worse than blowing your diet and then realizing you didn't even get much pleasure out of it. All those calories down the drain!

Create tradeoffs. If you're tempted to indulge in a favorite food, such as potato chips, force yourself to wait until after you've exercised. You might decide to trade ten minutes on the treadmill for one serving. This can serve to either motivate you to exercise for those ten extra minutes (if you really must have those chips) or it can motivate you to skip the chips if you're not willing to exercise.

Make up other trade-offs or games to play with yourself that will help you resist temptation and stay on track. If there's a food day at work then have a salad for dinner. If you know you'll be going out with friends at night then eat a light lunch. Strive for balance—if you overeat one day, undereat the next.

If you have a craving for a treat, it's okay to enjoy it as long as you don't overdo it. You can have one cookie, one small brownie, or one glass of soda instead of tons of everything. Remember to use moderation—you can eat anything you want, just not *everything* you want!

Remind yourself of your own personal motivators. Go back and review the motivators you entered in the personal plan you created in Chapter 1. Think hard about all the good reasons you don't want to gain weight. You might even be able to come up with a few more. This may help you stick to your resolution.

Develop a can-do attitude. Think of hunger pangs like a headache—unpleasant but bearable. Just because you're hungry or have a particular craving doesn't mean you have to cave in. Be tough and soldier through it. I'm sure you can think of other tough things you've had to bear. Remind yourself of your own inner strength. Also remember there are plenty of other desires you regularly resist—say, those cute shoes in the store window.

> "Strength is the capacity to break a chocolate bar into four pieces with your bare hands—and then eat just one of the pieces."
> Judith Viorst

Accept the bad days. I'm afraid we all have them! Just put them behind you and move on. Don't feel you can't excuse yourself for an occasional failure—losing or maintaining weight is hard work! Falling off the wagon for one day or even one week is not a total failure; it's only a setback.

When you have a bad period where you gave in to temptation, ask yourself what the reason was for not sticking with your plan. Be honest with yourself. Once you understand what's behind your temporary failure, you can address the barrier and overcome it.

Create graphs or charts to keep a record of your success. It may seem a little nerdy, but it works! Each day when you weigh yourself, jot down your weight. Take the entries over a period of time and enter them into a spreadsheet on your computer. Then create a graph from the data. Here's an example of a month I charted for my own weight:

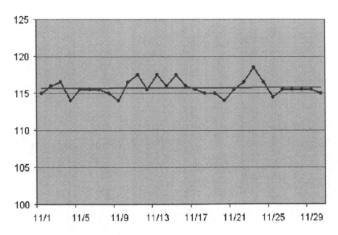

Daily Weight in November 2007
with trendline

As you can see, my weight went up or down a little each day, but that's to be expected. I actually ended the month at the same weight I began it with. Your goal is to keep your weight within the upper and lower bounds that you have set for yourself. When you can see the overall trend for how well you're maintaining your ideal weight, you'll feel motivated to keep it going. In my case, my weight started going up around November 21 (could it have been Thanksgiving week?), so I realized I needed to be more conscientious about my eating habits for a few days to bring my weight back within my desired range.

Graphing is also a useful aid when you're actually dieting. Seeing your progress over time will help you get past those periods when you may seem to be treading water or even going backwards a little. If your trend isn't going in the right direction, your chart will give you a warning so you can take action before it becomes a bigger problem. Maybe you can kick up your exercise program or cut back on your calories for a while until you get back on track.

Here's a chart that shows my progress when I was dieting many years ago:

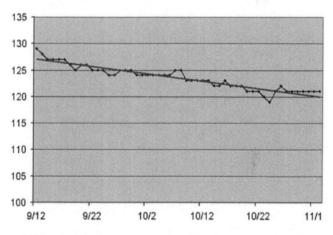

Daily Weight September - November 1999
with trendline

This chart was very motivational to me as I could see my steady progress. I could also see how close I was to achieving my final goal.

If you're not a computer whiz, just get some graph paper and do it by hand. The concept is the same, even if the chart isn't as fancy.

You can use the same technique with your waist measurement, your minutes of daily exercise, or whatever it is you want to track that's important to motivating you.

Work out with a friend. At times you may be tempted to blow off a workout, but it will be much harder to skip if you know someone is depending on you. Either your guilt or your sense of duty will come through to help you resist the temptation to quit. Once you are there and actually start working out, you'll be glad you made the effort—not just to support your friend, but to fulfill your commitment to yourself and your plan.

Sometimes gyms or YMCAs have programs that pair up people as exercise partners. Perhaps you have a neighbor who would like to walk with you regularly. Enlist your spouse or children if possible and exercise as a family. It's a great idea to instill healthy habits in your children at an early age. No matter who it is, you'll find yourself more motivated when you work out with a buddy.

Always carry an emergency food around with you when you're out. This could be a nutritious cereal bar, some hard candy such as a peppermint, or even a pack of gum. If you're away from home and you start to get hungry, you can use your emergency food to tide you over so you're not tempted to run in to the nearest candy store or fast food restaurant. This gives you control over how many calories you choose to consume.

At work, keep a stash of healthy food in your desk. Instead of turning to a vending machine for fattening candy bars or chips, have a cup of instant oatmeal (100 calories) or a low sugar granola bar (90 calories).

My workout buddies were shocked when I told them I carry Dove chocolates in my purse for emergencies. But remember, I'm not on a diet—I am merely maintaining my current weight. When I start to feel hungry, I'll allow myself one or two chocolates, which is all it takes to satisfy my craving. At 40 calories each, these treats fit into my personal eating plan. Having a chocolate not only helps me resist the temptation to stop and buy a high-calorie treat, but sometimes just knowing it's there if I want it is enough for me. I may tell myself I'll wait ten minutes before I indulge. Sometimes I've actually forgotten I wanted it by then as I get involved in my shopping or other activity.

Elvis loves Werther's butterscotch hard candies. I always keep a few in my purse for his emergency food when we're out together. He's usually satisfied with one piece of candy, which contains 22 calories. I'm sure we would have made a lot more trips to the bakery or ice cream shop if it weren't for my emergency supply.

Stay away from your eating buddies from your old "fat" times. If you have a friend with bad eating habits and you are tempted to overeat anytime you see her, control the situations when you're together. People tend to enjoy dining with others who share their food choices. This is basically the same principle as recovering alcoholics staying away from their drinking buddies to avoid situations where they may be tempted to start drinking again.

You don't have to give up your old relationships (assuming they were based on something more than having overeating in common). Instead of meeting your friend for lunch, dinner, or happy hour, try to think of a different type of get-together that doesn't focus on food. Maybe you could go to a play or a movie. Better yet, do something physically active together, such as roller-skating. You might be able to motivate her to improve her eating and exercising habits rather than you following her bad example.

Keep busy. When you're bored, you're more likely to

crave snacks. If you can keep yourself occupied, you'll be able to get your mind off of eating. A side benefit of keeping busy is that you just might use your time productively and accomplish something! For example, I like to bring a craft project, such as knitting a scarf, to family get-togethers. Not only does it keep my hands too busy to dip into the appetizers, but I have also produced many handcrafted items over the years.

Gardening is a hobby of mine that certainly keeps me busy. When I start pulling weeds or pruning rosebushes, I can end up spending hours in the garden and I forget all about snacking. Before I know it, Elvis is calling me to say it's dinnertime.

Another hobby I enjoy is reading. There's nothing like getting caught up in a good book to keep you from thinking about food.

Build a support group. It's great to have family or friends you can turn to when you're faced with temptation. If your spouse really supports your desire to be healthy and not gain weight, he or she is likely to provide encouragement when your resistance is low. Friends are usually great sources of inspiration. You can make it reciprocal—be sure to let them know they can call you for support any time.

Your support group can be helpful even when you're not in "crisis" mode. You might want to establish weekly meetings to compare progress and set goals. Sharing successes is hugely motivating. You can also pick up new strategies which have worked for others.

> "Eat only because you're hungry, not because you're not full."

My mother belongs to a weight loss group that meets weekly. Each member weighs in at the beginning of the meeting. If she has maintained or lost weight since the previous weigh-in, she receives loud cheers and applause from the other members. This is great motivation!

Plan your treats in advance. I can easily pass on a tempting dessert when I know I have a special treat to look forward to later, such as my favorite fat-free, sugar-free pudding with a scoop of Cool Whip. That satisfies me just as much as a calorie-dense slice of cheesecake or piece of pecan pie.

I love to eat late in the evening (I know, that's a diet no-no) so I plan ahead to either make some instant pudding or have ready-made single servings available. This snack is less than 200 calories, compared to over 700 for that piece of cheesecake.

I have found that on the rare occasions when I do give in and have dessert at dinner, I am just a little disappointed that I no longer have my late-night treat to anticipate. It kind of takes the fun out of the evening.

I mentioned using deferred gratification as a motivator in Chapter 1. This technique of planning treats for later can also help you resist an immediate temptation.

Eat healthy foods first. If you're at a dinner party or buffet reception, alter your portion sizes so that you have larger servings of healthy food and small tastes of the higher calorie items. When you fill up on salad (remember to go easy on the dressing and toppings), vegetables, or broth-based soup you won't be as tempted to overindulge on the pasta, bread, or fried chicken. Many times having just a taste of the forbidden foods will keep you from feeling deprived, while still keeping your calorie intake under control.

Keep it simple. Eliminate a high-calorie or high-fat food that has been a major part of your diet. This can help you resist temptation by removing the need for making any decisions about whether or not to even have any of the food. Once you get in the habit of absolutely *never* having this food, the temptation eases.

One suggestion for a food to eliminate completely is soda. You might also try eliminating all sweets or all starches (potatoes, pasta, bread, and rice). This is a somewhat drastic technique, but it has the advantage of simplicity. You are freeing yourself from the tiring responsibility of having to make choices on whether to eat something or how much of it to eat. You don't have to worry about calorie counting or maintaining a food diary.

Nibble throughout the day. This technique will keep you from getting too hungry at any time. If you let yourself get to the point where you feel deprived and absolutely ravenous, it's much harder to stay in control. You may find yourself eating everything in sight!

If you eat small amounts of healthy food frequently, you'll always have something in your stomach so you don't feel empty. This also helps to stabilize your metabolism so your body continues to burn calories at a higher rate.

Remind yourself of your success. You've managed to lose weight, so take pride in your accomplishment. Hang before and after photos of yourself on the refrigerator or keep them in your purse or car. When you're faced with temptation, take a look at how good your "after" version looks and you'll feel motivated to stay that way. I'm sure you don't want to go back to looking like your "before" picture.

In addition to looking better, you've probably made some improvements to your general health when you lost weight. It's likely your blood pressure is now lower or you have been able to reduce your diabetes medication. Keep these benefits in mind when you're tempted to backslide into old habits.

Reward yourself for resisting temptation with a non-food treat. Since you're denying yourself a food reward, you've earned a different kind of prize. When you're forming a new habit, associating some form of reward with the behavior will make the process much easier. The reward reinforces the positive behavior. I guess that's kind of like giving Elvis a pat on the head when he takes out the trash.

You can be creative and set up any kind of reward you can think of. For example, allow yourself time to browse your favorite websites, play your favorite video game, or watch a movie only after you've performed your daily dose of your "new habit" of eating healthy and turning down the bad foods.

Keeping track of your progress is also a form of reward, as it gives you a sense of control. Write down a list stating your progress. It could look something like this:

Day 1 – consumed less than 1,600 calories
Day 2 – exercised for 45 minutes
Day 3 – did 25 push-ups

Post your list somewhere in the house where other members of the family can see it, too. Making others aware of your accomplishments can be a valuable reward. The progress you list could be sticking to an eating plan, exercising regularly, or maintaining a certain weight.

Also try to reward yourself for meeting your interim goals. Make it a small reward for small increments, so the reward happens frequently. For example, if your goal was to work out three times per week, reward yourself with something small at the end of the week if you made it. Maybe you could give yourself permission to stay up late and watch a movie all the way to the end. How about buying yourself a CD of your favorite performer? Think of whatever reward is likely to motivate *you* (as long as it's not a food reward!).

Your homework assignment

1. Develop a strategy you will use to help you resist temptation, either by choosing one (or more) of the suggestions listed above, or by coming up with your own unique plan.
2. Enter your defense strategy in Section 3 of your custom plan.

Part Two

Where Are You?
Where Should You
Be?

Chapter 4

Your Ideal Weight

Let's take a look at what a healthy weight really means. You need to be objective about this, as many people don't view their own bodies realistically. Some women seem to always feel they are too heavy, no matter what friends (and the bathroom scale) may say. When these women see themselves in the mirror, they focus on any perceived flaws or bulges instead of seeing their true image, which usually includes both good and maybe not so good features.

On the other hand, some people seem to have an unrealistically high opinion about their body image and may be in denial about their true size and shape. I hate to say it, but in my experience, these people tend to be mostly men. Take my husband Elvis, for example. When he looks in the mirror, he sees a well-chiseled physique and a full head of hair.

What we need to do is look at weight objectively. There are several ways to determine your ideal weight. I'm going to warn you right now, this chapter will involve several tables, charts and calculations, but don't worry! I'll help you get through the process.

The first step is to see where you are right now. If you find yourself in a normal or even ideal range, congratulations! You can use the tips in this book to develop habits that will allow you to maintain your perfect weight for the rest of your life.

On the other hand, if you are not at the point you should be, you can also use these techniques to help you lose weight and become more physically fit. Your focus can be shifted to a maintenance program once you have reached your goal weight.

Healthy weight ranges are based on height, frame size (how large your bones are), and gender. To determine your body's frame size, measure your wrist with a tape measure and use the frame size chart in Table 4.1 below to determine whether you are small, medium, or large boned.

Table 4.1 - Frame Size Chart

	Women's Frame Size			Men's Frame Size
Height	**under 5'2"**	**5'2" to 5'5"**	**over 5'5"**	**over 5'5"**
Small-boned	wrist size less than 5.5"	wrist size less than 6"	wrist size less than 6.25"	wrist size less than 6.5"
Medium-boned	wrist size 5" to 5.75"	wrist size 6" to 6.25"	wrist size 6.25" to 6.5"	wrist size 6.5" to 7.5"
Large-boned	wrist size more than 5.75"	wrist size more than 6.25"	wrist size more than 6.5"	wrist size more than 7.5"

Now locate your height and frame size in Table 4.2 (for women) or Table 4.3 (for men) below to find the recommended weight range for you.

Table 4.2 - Height & Weight Table for Women

Height & Weight Table For Women			
Height	Small Frame	Medium Frame	Large Frame
4'9"	**99-108**	**106-118**	**115-128**
4'10"	**100-110**	**108-120**	**117-131**
4'11"	**101-112**	**110-123**	**119-134**
5'0"	**103-115**	**112-126**	**122-137**
5'1"	**105-118**	**115-129**	**125-140**
5'2"	**108-121**	**118-132**	**128-144**
5'3"	**111-124**	**121-132**	**131-147**
5'4"	**114-127**	**124-138**	**134-152**
5'5"	**117-130**	**127-141**	**137-156**
5'6"	**120-133**	**130-144**	**140-160**
5'7"	**123-136**	**133-147**	**143-164**
5'8"	**126-139**	**136-150**	**146-167**
5'9"	**126-139**	**139-153**	**149-170**
5'10"	**132-145**	**142-156**	**152-173**
5'11"	**135-148**	**145-159**	**155-176**

Elle Marie

Table 4.3 - Height & Weight Table for Men

Height & Weight Table for Men			
Height	Small Frame	Medium Frame	Large Frame
5'2"	128-134	131-141	138-150
5'3"	130-136	133-143	140-153
5'4"	132-138	135-145	142-156
5'5"	134-140	137-148	144-160
5'6"	136-142	139-151	146-164
5'7"	138-145	142-154	149-168
5'8"	140-148	145-157	152-172
5'9"	142-151	148-160	155-176
5'10"	144-154	151-163	158-180
5'11"	146-157	154-166	161-184
6'0"	149-160	157-170	164-188
6'1"	152-164	160-174	168-192
6'2"	155-168	164-178	172-197
6'3"	158-172	167-182	176-202
6'4"	161-176	170-186	180-207

Another way to determine if you are at an appropriate weight is to calculate your Quetelet Index, named after Adolphe Quetelet, who invented it in the mid-19th century. This is more commonly known as the body mass index or BMI. BMI is a reliable measure of body fat based on height and weight and applies to both men and women. The calculation is done by multiplying your weight in pounds by 703, then dividing the result by the square of your height in inches. The numbers used in the formula may seem somewhat arbitrary, but the reason they're needed is to convert American measurements of inches and pounds into metric equivalents (kilograms and meters). Mr. Quetelet was Belgian, so I suppose the metric system must have made sense to him.

Here's an example. Say you are 5'4" tall and weigh 130 pounds. Convert 5 feet and 4 inches to 64 inches. Calculate the square of 64, which is 4,096. Now multiply 130 pounds by 703, giving you 91,390. Dividing 91,390 by 4,096 results in a body mass index of 22.3.

> "A 2004 National Health and Nutrition Survey showed 2/3 of adults in the United States were overweight, and almost 1/3 were obese.[1]"

The body mass index isn't a good indicator of your body fat if you are an athlete or are heavily muscled. The calculation may show you are overweight, when you really are carrying those extra pounds in dense muscle tissue. It may also underestimate body fat in older persons or those who have lost muscle mass. Also keep in mind that the BMI is intended for adults and doesn't apply to children.

You can use Table 4.4 below to look up your BMI. Look for your height across the top of the table, then move down until you find the row closest to your weight. This will provide an approximate BMI value.

Elle Marie

Table 4.4 - Body Mass Index

Height (inches)	58	59	60	61	62	63	64	65	66	67	68	69	70	71	72	73	74
BMI	Body Weight (pounds)																
19	91	94	97	100	104	107	110	114	118	121	125	128	132	136	140	144	148
20	96	99	102	106	109	113	116	120	124	127	131	135	139	143	147	151	155
21	100	104	107	111	115	118	122	126	130	134	138	142	146	150	154	159	163
22	105	109	112	116	120	124	128	132	136	140	144	149	153	157	162	166	171
23	110	114	118	122	126	130	134	138	142	146	151	155	160	165	169	174	179
24	115	119	123	127	131	135	140	144	148	153	158	162	167	172	177	182	186
25	119	124	128	132	136	141	145	150	155	159	164	169	174	179	184	189	194
26	124	128	133	137	142	146	151	156	161	166	171	176	181	186	191	197	202
27	129	133	138	143	147	152	157	162	167	172	177	182	188	193	199	204	210
28	134	138	143	148	153	158	163	168	173	178	184	189	195	200	206	212	218
29	138	143	148	153	158	163	169	174	179	185	190	196	202	208	213	219	225
30	143	148	153	158	164	169	174	180	186	191	197	203	209	215	221	227	233
31	148	153	158	164	169	175	180	186	192	198	203	209	216	222	228	235	241
32	153	158	163	169	175	180	186	192	198	204	210	216	222	229	235	242	249
33	158	163	168	174	180	186	192	198	204	211	216	223	229	236	242	250	256
34	162	168	174	180	186	191	197	204	210	217	223	230	236	243	250	257	264
35	167	173	179	185	191	197	204	210	216	223	230	236	243	250	258	265	272
36	172	178	184	190	196	203	209	216	223	230	236	243	250	257	265	272	280
37	177	183	189	195	202	208	215	222	229	236	243	250	257	265	272	280	287
38	181	188	194	201	207	214	221	228	135	242	249	257	264	272	279	288	295
39	186	193	199	206	213	220	227	234	241	249	256	263	271	279	287	295	303
40	101	198	204	211	218	225	232	240	247	255	262	270	278	286	294	302	311
41	196	203	209	217	224	231	238	246	253	261	269	277	285	293	302	310	319
42	201	208	215	222	229	237	244	252	260	268	276	284	292	301	309	318	326
43	205	212	220	227	235	242	250	258	266	274	282	291	299	308	316	325	334

Once you have determined your BMI, look it up in Table 4.5 below to see if it is within the preferred (normal) range.

Table 4.5 - BMI Range

Category	BMI Range
Starvation	less than 15.0
Underweight	15.0 - 18.5
Normal	18.5 - 25.0
Overweight	25.0 - 30.0
Obese	30.0 - 40.0
Morbidly Obese	greater than 40.0

In our example, your BMI of 22.3 is excellent. Congratulations!

Your homework assignment

1. Calculate your ideal weight and/or your BMI and enter them in Section 4 of your custom plan.

Chapter 5

Your Eating Personality

You now know your recommended weight range and your current BMI. The next step is to learn about your own eating style or personality. Once you have identified your personal style, you can find ways to tailor an eating plan to meet your needs. Take this quiz to learn which general type of plan is best suited for your personality and habits. Check the box for each question that you would answer yes to.

Eating Personality Quiz

☐ 1.   Did you have a normal body weight when younger but slowly gained weight after age 30?

☐ 2.   Do you like to eat a lot of high-protein foods such as meat, cheese, eggs, and seafood?

☐ 3.   Have you found it easy to lose weight in the past?

☐ 4.   Are you a vegetarian?

☐ 5.   Do you lack the patience for counting calories or anything else?

☐ 6.   Can you commit to always reading food labels?

☐ 7.   Do you prefer to eat small frequent meals throughout the day instead of fewer heavier meals?

☐ 8.   Have you tried low-calorie diets yet were unsuccessful in losing weight?

☐ 9. Do you need an eating plan that requires little planning or thought?

☐ 10. Do you enjoy eating grains and vegetables?

☐ 11. Are you leery about eating foods with artificial ingredients?

☐ 12. Do you think of food as simply fuel for your body?

☐ 13. Do you have the discipline to keep a log of what you eat?

☐ 14. Is it easy for you to fast (for example, before taking a medical test)?

☐ 15. Do you dislike "diet" foods?

☐ 16. Do you have high cholesterol or a history of heart disease or gallbladder disease?

☐ 17. Do you have a slow metabolism?

☐ 18. Are you male?

☐ 19. Are you too busy to spend much time worrying about what you eat?

☐ 20. Is variety in your diet important to you?

☐ 21. Do you like to keep things simple?

☐ 22. Do you eat out more than 4 times per week?

☐ 23. Do you sometimes have food cravings (for starchy and/or sugary foods)?

Elle Marie

Scoring Instructions

Circle the numbers in the grid below that correspond to your "yes" answers. Find which category has the highest number of yes answers in order to find your eating personality. For fun and for easy reference, I've labeled each category with a representative animal. Don't be surprised if you resemble several different animals!

Deer	1	6	7	13	20	22
Lion	2	6	8	13	17	23
Gorilla	3	5	11	15	18	21
Rabbit	4	6	8	10	13	16
Koala	5	9	12	14	19	21

Here is more information about each eating personality. In the next chapter, I'll refer to these eating types and make recommendations especially tailored for each one.

The deer. If you answered yes to questions 1, 6, 7, 13, 20, and 22, a low-calorie diet is best for you. Let's call this eating personality a deer, since deer typically eat all day long, but tend to munch on low-calorie foods.

If you are a deer, you can eat almost any food you like, as long as you don't consume more than your allowable number of calories each day. However, if you overindulge early in the day, you must eat less later to compensate. A deer should become familiar with calorie counts of common foods, or keep a calorie guide handy. You will need to get in the habit of checking food labels for the number of calories per serving. You may need to keep a log of the foods you eat.

The deer's plan allows for great variety in your diet. It also lends itself to easy substitution of low-calorie foods for regular versions, allowing you to have a greater quantity of food so you feel satisfied.

Let's assume you're currently at the weight you plan to maintain. If you're a deer, you'll watch your calorie intake, so you need to know how many calories you can consume without gaining weight. Your current weight and activity level are the important factors to consider. To calculate your daily caloric allowance for maintaining your weight:

- If you are sedentary or inactive: Multiply your current weight in pounds by 13
- If you are moderately active: Multiply your weight in pounds by 15
- If you are very active: Multiply your weight in pounds by 17 to 19

For example, if you weigh 130 pounds and are moderately active, you can consume 1,950 calories (130 times 15 = 1,950) per day without gaining weight.

Look for the deer picture in Chapter 6 to see which strategies are especially geared toward deer eating styles.

The lion. If you answered yes to questions 2, 6, 8, 13, 17, and 23, a low-carbohydrate diet is probably best for you. We can call this diet type a lion, since lions are known for being high protein (meat) eaters.

As a lion, you need to limit the amount of high-carbohydrate foods you consume. High carbohydrate foods include bread, potatoes, pasta, rice, baked goods, and sweets. The lion needs to be familiar with carbohydrate counts in common foods. You may need to keep a log of the foods you eat to make sure you are not exceeding the allowable amount of carbohydrates. However, once you get used to identifying and learning to avoid the high-carb foods, there's not much to it. This is the eating plan you need if you tend to get food cravings. These cravings will usually go away after a week or two on this plan.

Use a general guideline of consuming no more than 60 to 80 grams of carbs daily.

In Chapter 6, the lion will guide you to the strategies suited to your eating personality.

The gorilla. If you answered yes to questions 3, 5, 11, 15, 18, and 21, a portion-control diet is best for you. I call this eating type the gorilla, not because real gorillas watch their portions, but because most people who fall into this category happen to be men. My husband, for example, is a gorilla.

You can eat whatever types of foods you enjoy, as long as you limit yourself to only small amounts. You may need to limit yourself to 3 meals a day, with little or no between-meals snacking. The big advantage to being a gorilla is that there is no need for preparing special meals or keeping a log of your food intake. If you're too busy or just don't want to be bothered with counting calories, carbs, or fat grams, this may be the best plan for you. You must be sure to avoid large portions, though, and try not to snack. Using small plates works for many people, as well as eating slowly and savoring each bite so you feel satisfied.

Look for the gorilla picture to help find the eating tips appropriate for you. You know, that kind of looks like Elvis.

The rabbit. If you answered yes to questions 4, 6, 8, 10, 13, and 16, you should try a low-fat eating plan. I call this eating personality a rabbit.

A rabbit's eating plan calls for limiting the number of grams of fat you consume. A low fat diet can help lower your risk of heart disease, since high amounts of saturated fat can raise the "bad" LDL cholesterol levels in your blood, which can increase the risk of heart disease. Just remember that a diet full of low fat foods is not automatically a low calorie, healthy diet. Soda, jellybeans, fat-free ice cream, and pretzels are all low in fat, but they aren't low in calories, especially if you're not careful about portion size.

Also keep in mind that reducing fat in your diet too dramatically can be unhealthy for certain individuals. If you are sedentary and overweight, a diet low in fat and high in carbohydrates can cause an increase of triglycerides (fat) in the blood and a decrease in the "good" HDL cholesterol, which actually protects against heart disease. A diet too low in fat may be deficient in important dietary nutrients, such as zinc, some B vitamins, and certain essential fatty acids that your body needs. You also need some fat in your diet in order to help your body absorb the fat-soluble vitamins A, D, E, and K, as well some compounds such as lycopene.

Use the calculations below to find your maximum number of fat grams to be consumed daily:

- If you are sedentary or inactive: Multiply your current weight in pounds by .4
- If you are moderately active: Multiply your weight in pounds by .5
- If you are very active: Multiply your weight in pounds by .57 to .63

These formulas assume that no more than 30% of your calories will come from fat. As an example, if your current weight is 130 pounds and you are moderately active, you can consume up to 65 grams of fat daily and still be able to maintain your weight. (130 times .5 = 65)

Look for the rabbit in Chapter 6 for your best tips.

The koala. If you answered yes to questions 5, 9, 12, 14, 19, and 21, an eating plan that limits certain foods will probably work best for you. You may have the type of personality that tends toward compulsiveness, so you need to build in controls for yourself. We'll call you a koala. After all, koalas only eat eucalyptus leaves, so their diet is very simple and limited.

You need to identify the "bad" foods and avoid them at

all times. No exceptions! Forbidden foods may include sweets, fried foods, and potato chips. If you avoid these foods, you can eat anything else you want. This means you don't have to count calories, carbohydrates, or fat grams. It simplifies your whole approach to eating, so you can focus on other things in your life. You never need to keep a log of the foods you eat.

You do need to make sure your selection of bad foods is comprehensive enough to make a difference. For example, if you currently drink 6 cans of regular soda each day (840 calories!), giving up that habit will make a huge difference. Giving up rice and pasta may work for you if those foods are currently a large part of your regular food consumption. If you only have pasta once a month, however, you need to find something else to avoid.

Be sure to look for the koala for the eating tips that are best for you.

Keep in mind these are very general categories of weight-maintenance plans. What works best for you may be to combine some elements of two or more plans. For example, I try to limit my overall calorie intake, without avoiding any particular food altogether. However, I choose low-fat and low-carb foods whenever I don't feel it compromises my enjoyment of the food I eat. I also watch my portion sizes. I guess that makes me a deerabbionilla hybrid. Find out what works for you, using your quiz results as a starting point.

Your homework assignment

1. Enter your eating type animal in Section 5 of your custom plan.

Part Three

Fill Up on Food Tips

Chapter 6

Eating Right for Your Type

To maintain your ideal weight, you must of course take control of your eating habits. But who wants to feel like they're on a perpetual diet? Dieting is hard work! You may have already been through some type of diet and exercise program to successfully reach your current weight, and you've probably had enough of diets. Or maybe you're close to the same weight you've always been (lucky you!) but now you're worried about your metabolism slowing down as you get older so you want to nip it in the bud before you start gaining. In either case, you need to learn how to keep from putting extra pounds on without feeling deprived.

No matter how motivated you are, you need some real-life strategies to help you develop healthy eating habits that work for *you*. I'm sure you've read books, magazine articles, and websites with lots of rules from "diet experts" on how to lose weight or simply keep the weight off. I know I have. But what really works for the long term?

The only way to find out is to experiment and discover which techniques will work for you. Understand your own individual likes and dislikes and work them into your plan. Obviously, you're just setting yourself up for failure if you choose a "cabbage soup diet" but you hate cabbage. (See Top 10 Worst Diets on next page.) However, if life just isn't worth living for you if you can't have chocolate, then you need to figure out how to allow chocolate in your eating plan, yet still be able to maintain an ideal weight.

Top 10 Worst Diets[1]

1. Caveman diet. Dine like the Flintstones on nuts, berries, fruits, vegetables, and meat. Also referred to as "prehistoric" Atkins—no grains allowed.
2. Sleeping Beauty diet. Zonk out on sedatives for a few days to lose weight. You can't binge while you're unconscious.
3. Cigarette diet. Cigarettes as dieting aids boosted Lucky Strike sales more than 200% in the 1920s with the catchy slogan, "Reach for a Lucky Instead of a Sweet."
4. Drinking man's diet. Drink your meals in this alcohol-based diet.
5. Cabbage soup diet. Eat all you want, as long as it's water and cabbage.
6. Grapefruit diet. First, you need to love grapefruit. Then, you have to stick to the diet for 21 days. Finally, you lose weight and learn to hate grapefruit.
7. Fletcher diet. Chew food 32 times but don't swallow. Spit it out, instead. Invented by Horace Fletcher in 1903, the idea is to absorb fewer calories while still enjoying the food's flavor. You may not be very popular at dinner parties.
8. The last chance diet. Starve yourself into thinness by drinking a protein concoction made from slaughterhouse leftovers that have been ground and flavored. It proved to be a dangerous diet in the 1970s.
9. Vinegar diet. The poet Lord Byron doused food with vinegar to quell his appetite. He lost more than 60 pounds.
10. Cheater's diet. Diet during the week; pig out on ice cream, burgers and beer on weekends.

I have compiled as many ideas as I could find for you to

consider. Many of them are strategies I use every day myself to manage my own weight. Some ideas were contributed by other people who have used them successfully. Others are just common sense and you may already be familiar with them. I'll admit right now that these are not all original ideas.

In some cases, these tips may contradict each other. What works well for one individual may not be helpful at all for another—in fact just the opposite technique will work. But each one of these suggestions can be used effectively by the right person.

In Chapter 5, you learned about your own personal eating style and preferences. Now I'll share with you some ideas that are especially suited to each type.

Let's start building your own personal eating plan. Choose which strategies you want to try out. If they work for you, make them part of your life. If they don't, try something else. But don't give up!

Substitute healthy foods. One of the most successful strategies for me is food substitution: replacing so-called "normal" foods with low-fat, low-calorie, or low-carb substitutes. Sometimes you can find foods that are low in all three categories! Diet or "lite" foods have come a long way over the years, and I think many of them now taste as good as the original.

I admit I have a sweet tooth. One of the foods I indulge in is sugar-free, fat-free pudding. You can get this in ready-to-eat 60-calorie snack cups, or you can use instant pudding mix and make it with skim milk (70 calories per serving). Since it is so low in calories, I allow myself two servings for a treat. Cheesecake and white chocolate are my favorite flavors, but you can find a large variety in most grocery stores.

I also like cottage cheese and I have found that the low-fat variety tastes just as good to me as whole fat, while saving 30 calories per 4 ounce serving. Skim milk can be used in place of 2% or whole milk to save lots of fat and calories. I always use skim milk in recipes that call for whole milk. I do try to make sure Elvis is not in the room at the time, though. He refuses to eat anything low fat and he believes he can tell the difference. Well, as I always say, what he doesn't know won't hurt him!

It's true some low-calorie foods don't taste exactly like the highly sugared originals. However, if you try these foods, you may discover you can develop a taste for them. Just give it a little time.

An example is unsweetened applesauce. When I first tried it, I thought it tasted pretty bland. However, after eating it regularly for a few weeks, I got used to the flavor and began to like it. When I accidentally had some regular applesauce some time later, it tasted much too sweet to me. I actually prefer the unsweetened variety now, which has 50 fewer calories per 4 ounce serving.

You can also get used to low-fat mayonnaise, fat-free cream cheese, 2% shredded cheese, and low-cal salad dressing. Keep in mind that some diet foods are an acquired taste that may take some time to adjust to. After all, you probably didn't like beer the first time you tried it, did you? Although actually I think Elvis did. Anyway, give food substitution a chance. It's an easy way to shave hundreds of calories from your food consumption each day.

Other substitutions I have made include:

- Five pieces of Melba toast instead of two slices of regular toast (savings of 60 calories)
- Sugar-free jam instead of regular jelly (savings of 44 calories per tablespoon)
- Unsweetened oatmeal with Splenda instead of regular oatmeal (savings of 50 calories)
- Light yogurt instead of regular (savings of 60 calories)

See Table 6.1 below for a comparison of other common diet foods to regular foods. The white rows contain information about regular foods and the shaded rows contain information about the recommended substitute.

Table 6.1 - Comparison of Normal Food to Substitutions

Food	Serving Size	Calories	Carbohydrate Grams	Fat Grams
Edy's Grand ice cream (Vanilla Bean)	½ cup	140	15	8
Blue Bunny personals light (Chocolate Raspberry Cheesecake)	½ cup	100	18	2.5
2 eggs	2 eggs	150	1	10
Egg Beaters	½ cup	60	1	0
Amber Bock	12 oz.	166	15	0
Bud Select	12 oz.	99	3	0
Regular instant pudding (made with whole milk)	½ cup	163	28	4.5
Sugar-free, fat-free instant pudding (made with skim milk)	½ cup	70	12	0
Regular potato chips	1 oz.	155	15	11
Baked potato chips	1 oz.	120	23	2
Regular mayonnaise	1 tbsp	90	0	10
Light mayonnaise	1 tbsp	40	0	4.5
Regular cottage cheese	4 oz.	110	3	5
2% fat cottage cheese	4 oz.	90	8	2
Fried chicken breast (battered, with skin)	6 oz.	442	15	22
Baked chicken breast (skinless)	6 oz.	275	0	6

Have a snack before dinner. If you eat something containing fat right before dinner, you may actually eat less during your meal. Try to keep the snack between 70 and 100 calories and make sure it contains healthy fats (no trans fats!). Nuts, for example, make a good before-dinner treat. A serving of 6 walnuts, 12 almonds, or 20 peanuts will have about 70 calories.

By eating some fat, you can fool your body into feeling satisfied sooner. Good fats stimulate the production of a fullness hormone (cholecystokinin, or CCK) that sends a signal to your brain that you've had enough to eat.

Experiment with sugar substitutes. There are many sugar substitutes on the market today that are used in all types of products. I personally prefer Splenda (sucralose), but Equal (aspartame), Sweet 'N Low (saccharin), and sorbitol are also very good and are nearly calorie free. By comparison, sugar contains 45 calories per tablespoon or 720 calories per cup, so this can make a big difference.

Today's sugar replacement products are nothing like those of ten years ago. You can use them in coffee, tea, or lemonade. You can bake and cook with them. I use them in all kinds of recipes and my family doesn't know the difference. (Please don't mention this to Elvis. I'm afraid if he knew I used Splenda in all my recipes, he'd decide he didn't like them anymore. Remember, he's a gorilla.)

Try more low-calorie foods. Take a tour of your local grocery store and see what it has to offer in the way of low-calorie foods. Don't be afraid to try something new.

For many years, I hesitated to try Egg Beaters because somehow I had the idea they were "fake" eggs. One day I saw an advertisement that claimed they were 99% real eggs. That claim made me curious, so the next time I went grocery shopping, I examined the label and discovered that Egg Beaters are actually made from egg whites, with a tiny amount of vitamins and seasoning added. They have less than half the calories of whole eggs, but they *are* real eggs. I now use them in omelets and various recipes regularly.

One easy way to save lots of fat and calories is to use a cooking spray such as Pam instead of cooking oil. This trick will literally save you hundreds of calories. One tablespoon of olive oil has 120 calories and 14 grams of fat. Cooking spray has almost none of either.

I love rice cakes. They come in many flavors, both salty and sweet, so they can be substituted for salty snacks like potato chips or for sweet snacks like cookies. I've even seen main dish recipes using rice cakes as a substitute for tortillas or bread.

Another favorite food of mine is sugar-free yogurt. Some varieties have as little as 40 calories per 4-ounce serving. This is a healthy, satisfying snack that's good for you but doesn't pack on the pounds. The calcium in yogurt is an added bonus for women, who need about 1,000 mg per day.

Top 10 Tastiest Low-Calorie Foods

1. Blue Bunny personal light ice cream
2. Yoplait light yogurt
3. Jell-O pudding with Cool Whip on top
4. Morningstar Chik Patties
5. Cheesy popcorn cakes
6. Strawberries with Splenda on top
7. Mixed veggies with light butter and garlic herb seasoning
8. Reduced sugar granola bars
9. Baked potato chips
10. Special K cereal

Enjoy lower-calorie drinks. What you drink is just as important for maintaining your weight as what you eat. Most people drink about 20% of their daily calorie intake, so this can make a big difference.

Many diets recommend cutting out alcohol completely, but that may not be realistic for everyone, especially for socially active people. If you want to drink on social occasions, try to find drinks that are lower in calories.

Beer may be the biggest culprit when it comes to alcohol causing weight gain. I'm sure you've heard of the dreaded beer belly! In general, beers with less alcohol will be less fattening. Of course, if drinking those beers means you'll have twice as many, then the math no longer works in your favor.

You may want to consider Guinness. Although it is often seen as a fattening brew, it actually has a surprisingly average 126 calories per serving. In general, the biggest offenders are dark beers, but remember that you can easily hit 500 or more calories once you start drinking more than two bottles of almost any brand of beer.

Try to avoid Anchor Porter, one of the highest-calorie American beers (209 calories per 12-ounce serving), and McEwans Scottish Ale, one of the highest-calorie imported beers (295 calories). If you don't mind light beers, Pabst Extra Light Low Alcohol has only 67 calories per 12-ounce serving, and Molson Light jumps to 82 calories for the same amount. Anheuser Busch Michelob Ultra comes in at 95 calories per standard serving.

For mixed drinks, try ordering diet soda with a splash of whatever alcohol you like, rather than ordering a standard mixed drink. That way, you can still enjoy the taste of the drink, but at a fraction of the alcohol so there aren't as many calories. Or consider a Bloody Mary, a highball, or a Manhattan, with each containing an average calorie count in the mid 100s for a standard serving.

What about liquors? Again, you can generalize that the amount of calories in liquor is directly related to its alcohol content. On average, one fluid ounce of vodka, whiskey, or brandy at 50% alcohol (100 proof) will deliver 82 calories each. Schnapps is a bit higher-calorie at around 95 calories per fluid ounce. Of course, the most calories come from the sweet liquors, or liqueurs. An ounce of crème de menthe, for instance, registers an average of 125 calories.

If wine is your preferred drink, you should avoid Ruby Port, which has 185 calories in a 4-ounce glass. On the other hand, white zinfandel tends to be one of the safest bets with a modest 80 calories. Other good choices are Chardonnay, at around 90 calories, or Chablis, at 85 calories. Although calorie counts aren't listed on wine bottles, the alcohol content is listed. You can assume that the more alcohol a wine has the more calories it will have.

If you normally drink a lot of regular soda, switching to

diet soda can save an incredible number of calories. Four 12-ounce servings of regular soda have 560 calories and no nutritive value. If you can get used to the taste of diet soda, you will find that the pounds will drop off and stay off. Since there are 3,500 calories in a pound, you could lose about a pound a week by making this one change. If you're not ready to completely make the transition from regular to diet soda, how about mixing them half and half? After a while, you can increase the proportion of diet soda until you're used to the taste and you can completely eliminate the regular soda.

There are many tasty protein and diet shakes on the market today. Try them as a substitute for breakfast or lunch occasionally. They're full of nutrition and have fewer calories than a regular meal.

Watch your portion size. If you're careful about portions, you can eat whatever type of food you like. If you want to lose weight without counting calories, just eat the same food you normally do, but cut each serving in half. This technique is great for busy people or people like Elvis who just don't want to be bothered with food diaries or calorie counters.

This type of eating plan can also be used for weight maintenance, but it does take some discipline. If you don't want to weigh or measure your food, you need to learn how to judge the appropriate serving size. One easy way is to always read the labels on packaged foods. Serving size will be listed so you can judge whether you should eat the whole package or only one-fourth of it.

Another way to determine portion size is to compare your food to common, everyday objects. For example, a standard 3-ounce serving of meat or fish is about the size of a deck of cards. A medium portion of fruit is about the size of a tennis ball. Half a bagel the size of a hockey puck represents one serving from the grain food group. One and a half ounces of cheese is about the size of two dominoes. In general, one cup is about the size of your fist or a baseball, so if you're estimating how much pasta or rice you're having, use this as a guide.

At meals, serve yourself appropriate portions, and then put any extra food away so you won't be tempted to have second helpings. Just remember, if you're on a portion-controlled eating plan, you can eat anything you want as long as you don't eat too much of it.

Never eat out of the bag (chips) or box (cookies). This is a sure way to sabotage your portion control. Instead, measure out how much you plan to eat into a bowl or dish, and then put the bag away. If you're going to have a dessert, cut the cake or pie into smaller pieces before serving.

Elvis is a strong believer in portion size. He thinks that as long as you eat less food, it doesn't matter which foods you eat. So according to his way of thinking, you could eat a bowlful of chocolate and it would have the same effect as a bowlful of lettuce. After all, the portion sizes are the same.

While I might have a large salad with light dressing for dinner (at about 200 calories and 10 grams of fat), he'll have a hamburger (300 calories, 12 grams of fat) with cheese (100 calories, 7 grams fat) and some French fries (260 calories, 14 grams of fat). He'll make sure his plate has the same basic amount of food on it as mine, but he makes very different choices. Surprisingly, he's not losing weight!

However, watching your portion sizes is important, especially if you want to avoid calorie counting. If you do want to be able to eat whatever types of food you prefer, you'll have to go easy on the ones that are calorie-dense. Generally, the more moisture content a food has, the lower it is in calories (think of watermelon or lettuce). Denser, lower moisture foods such as dried fruit are much higher in calories, ounce per ounce. However, as long as you have small portions, even pasta in Alfredo sauce is okay.

Keep a food log. This can be a lot of work, but it is also very effective in helping you manage your food consumption. Counting calories is one sure way to make sure you don't gain weight. Most people underestimate the number of calories they consume each day by about 25%. This can easily happen by forgetting to count a few nibbles here and there, not including calories from beverages, or missing the extra calories in dressings, sauces, or toppings.

A basic way of tracking your food intake is to 1) list everything you eat; 2) look up or estimate the number of calories in each item; and 3) keep a running total for the day. Once you hit your pre-determined limit, don't allow yourself to eat anything else that day.

I got into this habit many years ago when I decided I needed to lose 20 pounds. I started logging in each item of food I ate, along with its calorie count. I allowed myself no more than 1,500 calories per day on Saturday through Thursday. On Fridays, when Elvis and I eat out to celebrate the end of the workweek, I allowed myself up to 1,800 calories. This strategy helped me lose those 20 pounds, but I kept up with the log even after I reached my goal weight and went on a maintenance plan. I raised my daily limit to 1,800 calories, but I was afraid if I didn't carefully track everything that went into my mouth, I'd regain the weight I had worked so hard to lose. I was finally able to let go of this habit after about six months, but it's still a tool I use occasionally.

When I was keeping a food diary, I became very familiar with the serving sizes and calorie counts of common foods. It was very enlightening to learn that some foods I thought were good diet foods actually were higher in calories than I expected. On the other hand, I learned about great nutritious foods that were low in calories. For many months, I carried around a pocket calorie counter (which Elvis gave me for Christmas, that sweetheart!) until I had pretty much memorized it. I also became very adept at reading nutrition labels and looking up nutrition information on websites.

Counting calories may be enough for you to stay on track with your weight. However, you may also want to track your carbohydrate or fat grams. In that case, add columns to your food log for these amounts and fill them in for each item you consume. For your convenience, I have included sample food logs in Appendix B. I recommend this strategy for lions who are trying to limit their carbohydrate intake. You can buy a purse-sized book with carbohydrate amounts listed for common foods.

Yet another way of using a food log is to calculate the proportions of carbohydrates and protein that you consume. This is recommended for low-carb eating plans. In addition to keeping your total calorie intake below your recommended amount, you should try to keep your carbohydrates to 40% or less, and your protein intake at 40% or more. This leaves approximately 20% of your calories from fat. You can use the spreadsheet provided on my website, or create your own using the formulas provided in Appendix B. Enter in each food you eat, along with the number of grams of carbs and protein.

Maybe you're interested in keeping track of your fiber intake. Many Americans do not consume enough fiber. The recommended amount is 25 grams per day for women and 30 grams per day for men. You can add another column to your calorie counter for tracking grams of fiber.

Another easy way of tracking any of those amounts is to use an online tracker. One great free website is www.fitday.com. When you enter the foods you eat it will automatically track your calories, fiber, protein, carbohydrates, and even vitamins. You can also use this website to log physical activity and estimate how many calories you have burned off in each one.

Lighten up your foods. Look for ways to make your favorite foods healthier, such as using less butter, dressing, or rich sauces. When eating out, ask for your salad dressing on the side and use it for dipping, rather than drenching the whole salad. I'm afraid that's how Elvis likes his salad – drenched in about half a bottle of dressing. At a restaurant, he'll have dressing on his salad, and then ask for additional dressing on the side which he pours on top. I call it his "salad soup". But he believes he's eating healthy, because after all, it's just a salad.

In our local newspaper, there's a column in the food

section where the food editor takes an ordinary recipe and then modifies it to reduce fat, carbs, and calories. It's amazing what you can do with light sour cream, light mayonnaise, and low-fat rolls. Simple substitutions can save lots of calories without noticeably affecting the taste or texture. I've tried many of these recipes with great results.

You can reduce the amount of fat in corn breads and cakes by substituting unsweetened applesauce for part or all of the oil in the recipe. Use canola or peanut oil instead of shortening or lard (does anyone still use lard?) for fried items. Better yet, sauté food in cooking spray instead of frying.

Top 10 Tastiest Low-Fat Foods

1. Lobster
2. Any kind of wine
3. Blueberries
4. Frosted flakes
5. Jelly beans
6. Angel food cake
7. Melba toast with cream cheese
8. English muffin
9. Pretzels
10. Artichokes

Add more protein to your diet. The average Western diet consists of 49% carbohydrates, 35% fat, and 16% protein. By contrast, the typical caveman diet contained 35% more protein than modern man. I bet you never heard of an overweight caveman!

Studies have found that increasing the protein content of meals leads to an increased level of the fullness hormone PeptideYY, when compared to high fat or high carbohydrate meals[2]. This hormone will make you feel more satisfied and help keep you from overeating. On the other hand, a diet high in carbs can leave you constantly hungry.

Here are some facts about protein:

- Protein requires 25% more energy to digest than carbs or fat.

- Unlike carbs or fat, the body doesn't store protein.
- Protein stimulates muscle growth—each pound of muscle burns 35 calories/day, while a pound of fat burns merely two calories daily.

Top 10 Tastiest Low-Carb Foods

1. Shrimp
2. Whipped cream
3. Cream cheese
4. Macadamia nuts
5. Mushrooms
6. Steak
7. Eggs
8. Butter
9. Avocados
10. Strawberries

Use smaller plates. You may have heard this tip before, but now research has proven that using smaller plates and smaller bowls can help you lose weight. In our society, not only are food portions huge, these super-sized meals are usually served on large plates. One of the easiest and most direct ways to control portions is to control what we choose to serve our food on. Smaller portions mean fewer calories, which translates into weight loss or maintenance.

New plates you find in stores are typically about 11 inches in diameter. However, if you look at antique plates from earlier times, you'll find they are only eight inches across. If you switch to plates of a similar size as those our grandparents and great-grandparents used, you may find it easier to maintain a weight closer to that of earlier generations.

Not only do smaller plates encourage you to eat less, but the way you place the foods on your plate can also help you cut calories. Think of dividing up your meals this way: use 1/4 of the plate for protein, 1/4 for carbohydrates, and the remaining 1/2 for vegetables (remember that vegetables are the lowest-calorie food group). This is an easy way to have a portion- and calorie-controlled meal.

This approach also works with glasses. Using tall, thin glasses gives the illusion of drinking more than using a shorter, wider glass that may actually hold more liquid. If you're drinking water, unsweetened tea, or diet soda, don't worry about it. But if you're drinking anything else, including fruit juice or alcoholic beverages, keep this tip in mind.

Eliminate *all* sweets. This may seem drastic, but it has two major advantages: 1) it's very simple to understand and 2) it works! Just get into the habit of *never* eating anything sweet. This includes cake, pie, cookies, ice cream, and candy. Yes, it's hard, but the easy part is not having to track your calories or fat grams.

Maybe you have a candy bar habit that is causing you to gain unwanted pounds. Although you may feel you need to eat that candy bar, your need is probably emotional, not physical. Keeping in mind that it can take 30 days to break an old habit or develop a new habit, try going "cold turkey" from your candy bars for 30 days. After that, it will be ingrained as part of your lifestyle.

Personally, I don't think this technique would work for me. It would require too much sacrifice for me to stick with it. Not every technique is for every individual, so choose the ones that make sense to you. Remember to use your animal type as a guide.

Carmello M. decided he needed to lose weight after seeing his wife Mary lose 60 pounds, but he didn't want to count calories or follow a strict meal plan. His approach was to reduce his portion sizes and eliminate what he calls the six "Cs" from his diet—cookies, cake, chocolate, cola, candy, and chips. To replace these foods, he started eating more vegetables and actually began to appreciate them. He also began exercising, starting out with short walks and working up to longer distances and brisker paces. Using this eating and exercise plan, Mello was able to lose 50 pounds and has kept them off. His cholesterol level also improved dramatically, allowing him to reduce his medications to only two pills a day.

Eliminate starchy foods. This food group includes pasta, rice, potatoes, and bread. Think of these as your "red-light foods" and respond to them just as you would to a red light—STOP. Since these foods are probably difficult for you to resist, you may find that completely eliminating them from your diet is the best way to succeed. After about two weeks of avoiding high-carbohydrate foods, you'll start to lose your craving for them.

Catherine V. used this approach successfully. She decided she wanted to lose about 20 pounds she had picked up over the years, but didn't want to have to "work" at it. She didn't have time to calculate calories or carbs intake or to plan special meals. So she just decided one day to stop eating starchy food. She gradually dropped the weight and has been able to keep it off ever since. She is now so used to skipping pasta and pizza that she doesn't even think about it anymore. And she loves her trim figure!

Eat three meals a day. This means sticking to only three meals with no between meal snacking. This way, you only need to be careful about what you eat three times each day, resulting in fewer decisions to make and a simpler life. In combination with portion control, this may be all you need to maintain your weight for life.

If you need to lose weight, you might want to try this approach, but with only two meals a day. If you are a morning person, eat breakfast and lunch, then stop eating for the rest of the day. If you're more of a night owl, eat lunch and dinner. Either way, avoid between meal treats and don't go overboard on meals.

Elaine V. tried this approach when nothing else seemed to work for her. She ate breakfast, then a late lunch. Once she was finished eating her lunch meal, she was through eating for the day. She dropped 15 pounds quickly using this strategy.

Be a grazer. Eat small amounts of food throughout the day. This strategy has the advantage of making you feel satisfied all day long. If you can avoid feeling hungry, you are less likely to overeat. You do need to be careful to have small, low-calorie snacks and you also need to have small portions at mealtime in order for this to be effective.

Small, frequent meals will help keep your metabolism revved up, thereby burning more calories overall. Try to include some protein for each snack and meal to have the most impact on your metabolism.

On the other hand, when you allow too much time between meals, your metabolism will slow down to compensate for what it perceives to be starvation mode. When you finally do eat, your body will want to hold on to every calorie to conserve its energy.

Your homework assignment

1. Select four - five eating tips that you think will work for you. Use your animal type as a guide for which ones are most likely to suit your personality and eating style.
2. Enter your eating strategies in Section 6 of your custom plan.
3. After two weeks, select two more ideas to try. Discard any of the earlier ones that haven't worked for you.
4. Continue gradually trying out the suggestions that appeal to you until you have hit on the most effective combination.

Chapter 7

Eating Tips for Everyone

There are many eating strategies that may be appropriate for anyone, regardless of your eating personality. In this chapter, I've put together more ideas for you to try.

Read on and discover the combination of strategies that can work for you, yet are easy (or at least bearable) for you to live with. Incorporate them into your regular habits and you'll find you have developed your own unique lifestyle of staying slim and healthy.

This is how to avoid feeling that you are continually on a diet, being forced to make sacrifices every day. When you're dieting, you have to expend a significant amount of energy focusing on what, when, and how much you eat, maybe even to the point of obsession. That might be acceptable for a limited period of time, but certainly not for the rest of your life.

So continue building your personal eating plan by adding more ideas from the list below.

Make small changes. Elvis likes to drink a scotch and have a handful of pretzels when he comes home from work. I guess you could call that his before dinner appetizer. One day he decided he should stop doing that every day so he could drop a few pounds after the holidays. He told me about his plan and

I was very supportive. I figured he would save about 400 calories each day, which would begin to add up and he would start slimming down. However, after several days, I noticed he was still having a scotch with pretzels each day. I asked him about his plan to stop this habit and he replied, "I said I wasn't going to do it *every* day." I guess that means that every once in a while, he'll skip it. That may not be a big change, but I suppose it's a step in the right direction.

Other small changes might include cutting down on regular soda (or replacing it with diet soda), using artificial sweetener instead of sugar in your coffee or tea, or skipping dessert. Think about your regular eating patterns and try to come up with ways to save a few calories. Over time, little things can add up to make a big difference.

Once when Elvis and I were visiting our state capitol building, we stopped in the café for a snack. I chose baked potato chips and a diet soda. He chose Fritos and a 16-ounce regular soda. While on the surface our snacks looked equivalent, he actually consumed 620 more calories and 36 more fat grams! When I examined the label on the bag of Fritos, I realized the bag actually contained four servings, at 160 calories per serving, totaling 640 calories. His soda was an additional 190 calories. My baked chips had only 210 calories and 3.5 grams of fat and my diet soda had no calories or fat at all. That just goes to show that making small changes in your food choices can have a big impact.

Eat slowly. Maybe over the years you've fallen into the habit of eating quickly. If you're a new mom, you may find yourself shoveling down anything you can get when you have a quick break from your baby duties. Or maybe you have a high-pressure job with few breaks and 24x7 responsibilities. There are lots of reasons for being too busy and rushed to take the time to eat slowly, but you know it's not healthy for you. It's also difficult to really enjoy your food when you just gulp it down in a hurry.

A better approach is to eat slowly and savor your food in small bites. This is better for your digestion and makes it easier to control portions. Research shows people eat approximately

67 fewer calories per meal when they slow down their pace[1]. If you slow down the pace for all three meals, you'll save 200 daily calories. Since it takes time (about 20 minutes) for your brain to receive the message that your stomach is full, slowing down allows you to know when you've had enough to eat.

Put your fork down between bites and thoroughly chew each mouthful before picking up your fork again. I am in the habit of cutting my food using my knife in my right hand and my fork in my left. After I cut a piece of food, I transfer the fork to my right hand and then spear the piece with my fork and eat it. This drives Elvis crazy. He considers it very inefficient. He prefers to eat European style, where the left hand uses the fork (assuming you're right-handed). Yes, it's quicker and more efficient, but who's in a hurry?

However, we can learn something from European countries, where meals are generally much more leisurely than in the U.S. By taking our time, we'll get more pleasure out of dining. It can be a social occasion rather than just a routine, necessary activity.

Another advantage of eating slowly is that you won't be the one who has to sit and wait for everyone else. I've observed quick eaters get bored when they're through with their meal in five minutes, but are required by good manners to sit politely while others finish. It's a lot less boring to be on the other end, where everyone else is waiting for you. The ideal situation, of course, is for everyone to eat slowly, enjoying their food and their companions, and to finish up at the same time.

If you don't have the time for a leisurely meal, at least sit down and eat to truly appreciate the food. Never eat standing up! If you do, you won't feel like you've even had a meal, and will probably feel the urge to eat again before long. When you're eating, try to focus on enjoying the food instead of multi-tasking. If you eat while watching television (as 66% of Americans do), working at your desk, or driving in your car, you'll be distracted from your meal. When you're distracted, you consume more food and feel less satisfied.

Fill up on fiber. Soluble fiber, found in grains, beans, and the pulp of fruits and vegetables, slows down your digestive process because it is digested by bacteria rather than stomach acid and enzymes. This keeps food in your stomach longer so you don't feel hungry. Soluble fiber absorbs cholesterol to prevent it from entering your bloodstream, which can help prevent heart disease. Fiber absorbs water and makes you feel fuller. It's also great for your digestion. Adding more fiber to your diet will curb your appetite and help flush calories out of your body.

A recent study indicates that higher fiber content in a meal increases levels of the satiety hormone cholecystokinin, the same hormone released when fats are eaten[2]. Scientists believe this hormone may be the chemical messenger that signals the brain when the body is getting full.

I like to get more fiber in my diet by eating plain instant oatmeal with ground flaxseed added. For only a little more than 100 calories, it's a satisfying breakfast with lots of fiber. I love the nutty taste of flaxseed and I add it to many foods, such as cottage cheese, yogurt, and applesauce. See Table 7.1 below to get some ideas for high fiber foods you may enjoy.

Try to get your necessary amount of daily fiber. Experts recommend 14 grams of fiber for every 1,000 calories consumed. That adds up to about 25 grams for women and 30 grams for men. By eating foods high in fiber, you're naturally going to be eating healthier, since fiber is mostly found in fruits, vegetables, and grains. If you fill up on fiber-rich foods, you won't be tempted to eat less healthy foods, such as potato chips.

Elle Marie

Table 7.1 - High Fiber Foods

Apple with skin	3.9 grams/1 medium
Artichoke hearts	4.4 grams/half cup
Blackberries	7.2 grams/cup
Bran cereal	10 grams/half cup
Broccoli	2.6 grams/half cup
Brussels sprouts	3.4 grams/half cup
Carrot	2.3 grams/1 average
Corn on the cob	2.9 grams/small ear
Kidney beans	4.5 grams/half cup
Lima beans	6.6 grams/half cup
Oatmeal	4 grams/cup
Orange	3.1 grams/1 medium
Pear	2.5 grams/1 medium
Peas	5.2 grams/half cup
Popcorn	2.8 grams/3 cups popped
Potato	3.8 grams/1 small
Prunes	11 grams/cup
Pumpkin seeds	3.9 grams/1 ounce
Raisins	3.9 grams/half cup
Refried beans	6.7 grams/half cup
Spinach	2 grams/half cup
Strawberries	3.9 grams/1 cup
Sweet potato	3.4 grams/1 small
Whole wheat bread	3.9grams/2 slices

Use spices generously. It's amazing how good plain vegetables can taste with a little low-fat margarine and some garlic herb seasoning. Since spices have a negligible amount of calories and add lots of flavor, you can use as much as you like. You can shake convenient spice blends on meat or vegetables, or you can use exotic spices in various recipes (see Appendix C - Recipes). Replace high-fat gravies and sauces with seasoning and you will save hundreds of calories and fat grams, while still enjoying flavorful dishes. You do need to be careful about adding little extras that may not seem to make a big difference but are high in calories, such as nuts or sunflower seeds.

This is a good suggestion for people concerned with maintaining their weight, but who still have to prepare meals for others who want to eat with more variety in their diets. I guess I'm talking about most wives and mothers here. You'll find your family will enjoy Chinese, Mexican, Indian, Italian, and other ethnic recipes which can be very flavorful but don't have to be high in calories.

Stretch your meals with filler foods. Maybe there's one food you really like that has very few calories. If so, you can eat a lot of that food as a filler to provide more satisfaction at your meals. Filling up this way will give you a greater quantity of food to eat, so you will feel more full.

> *"The average daily food intake of adults rose by about 300 calories between 1985 and 2000[3]."*

An example of this is pickles, especially the dill variety. This is one of Elvis's favorite foods. He'll eat a plateful of dill pickles with his lunch and he'll feel like he had a big meal, while actually consuming very few calories. How about lettuce? Two cups of lettuce contain only 15 calories, so you can basically eat as much as you like. One medium stalk of celery has only 6 calories. Many other vegetables are very low in calories, too. By increasing your quantity of healthy, low-cal foods, you can eat smaller amounts of other foods and still enjoy a variety of tastes.

Eat soup every day. Here is an easy way to reduce your calorie intake without feeling like you're making a sacrifice: eat a bowl of soup at least once a day. Nutritious, low-salt soups will provide nutrition, fill you up, and help flush waste from your body.

Studies have shown that people who eat a serving of soup daily consume 20% fewer calories than those who don't eat soup[4]. Homemade soup is best, but canned soups are fine if you prefer their convenience. Broth-based soups are lower in calories than creamy soups, but as long as you're careful about your portion size, either is fine. You're more likely to make this a regular habit if you choose soups you like.

I enjoy having instant soup for lunch each day. My favorite flavors are Spring Vegetable (45 calories), Hearty Chicken Noodle (70 calories), and Tomato (90 calories). I eat the hot soup first, which forces me to eat slowly. By the time I start eating the rest of my lunch, I'm already beginning to feel satisfied.

Eat more at night. Don't believe everything you've heard about eating at certain times of the day, or having a certain number of meals and snacks each day. If you're not a morning person and don't care to eat a large breakfast, then don't! What's important is what feels right to you.

I have never been a morning person. Or, as Elvis puts it, in the morning I'm not a person. When I wake up, it's all I can do to drag myself out of bed and get ready to face the day. Taking the time to prepare and eat breakfast would just mean I'd have to get up even earlier. So for my entire life, I've either skipped breakfast or eaten a very small, light meal. If I listened to the diet experts and ate a more substantial meal, I'd be adding several hundred calories to my daily diet, without getting much enjoyment from it. My philosophy is to make the calories count. Since there are a limited number of calories I can consume each day and still maintain the weight I want, I intend to thoroughly enjoy each one of them.

Although breakfast doesn't tempt me, I do love to eat in the evening. I regularly have a bedtime snack. When I mentioned this to friends I work out with, they responded with a loud collective gasp. They were absolutely horrified and could not believe that this habit wasn't packing on the pounds. I do limit myself to 200 calories or less for my evening snacking. Skipping breakfast seems to offset these calories, so somehow it comes out even. This tip can work for anyone, but is especially recommended for deer and rabbits.

Eat more early in the day. I realize not everyone is like me.

Many people really enjoy eating breakfast. As long as your total calorie count is within the recommended amount for your weight, you can consume those calories either early in the day or later. It's a matter of personal preference.

You may have heard the expression "Breakfast like a king, lunch like a prince, and supper like a pauper." I know a lot of folks who have been successful in maintaining their weight by following a guideline of eating more heartily early in the day, and then cutting off all food after 7:00 pm. This approach does work for many people. An advantage is the simplicity of having a hard and fast rule for yourself. With a firm cut-off time, you don't need to keep making decisions about whether or not to have one more snack. That's why this tip is especially recommended for gorillas, who like to keep things simple.

If you want to try out this strategy, make sure you don't skip breakfast. Studies have shown that people who don't eat breakfast often end up consuming more calories later in the day[5]. If you are more of a morning person who tends to be hungry as soon as you get up, you are likely to be starving if you don't have your breakfast. These hunger pangs could lead you to abandon your eating plan and overeat later.

The human body follows a circadian rhythm in digesting and utilizing food, meaning the same foods eaten at breakfast and lunch are processed differently than when eaten at dinner. Although this doesn't seem exactly logical to me, some studies have shown that when you eat your daily protein and fat at breakfast you tend to lose weight and have more energy; however, eating the same things at dinner can increase tendencies toward weight gain[6]. Erica G., a young woman I know, was able to lose 20 pounds by eating the same foods as always, but at earlier times of the day. This technique does work for some people and is definitely worth a try, especially if you're a gorilla.

Enjoy a limited indulgence. Allow yourself one small treat each day. This can be whatever food appeals to you. It could be a narrow slice of cake, a handful of pretzels, or a small serving of ice cream. If you allow yourself at least a small portion of your favorite food, you can avoid feeling deprived.

Otherwise that feeling of deprivation can build up and eventually lead you to overindulge.

Just knowing you can have a treat if you choose to will help you maintain your healthy eating habits. Remember there are still limits. If you allow yourself a large order of French fries on a daily basis, for example, don't expect to maintain your ideal weight.

Indulge your pickiness. What I mean by this is to only choose to eat food that truly appeals to you. For example, the idea of fat or gristle in meat or chicken is very unappetizing to me. I will cut off anything that resembles fat from my chicken or beef. Why should I eat something and consume the calories if I'm not going to really enjoy it? In fact, why would I eat something that I had to force myself to get down?

I also won't eat shrimp that has not been properly de-veined. While shrimp is an excellent, healthy food (a serving of five large shrimp has 40 calories, 1/2 gram of fat and less than 1/2 gram of carbohydrates), the thought of eating the "vein" disgusts me. After all, it's really just a euphemism for intestine, and we all know what's inside of intestines! Even if the shrimp has been properly cooked and there is no danger of bacterial infection, the idea of eating shrimp feces simply turns my stomach.

Now I'm not talking about spitting out food once it's in your mouth. I'm just recommending that you go ahead and pick off the sausage topping on your pizza if it doesn't appeal to you. Don't eat your piecrust if you don't like it. Food is supposed to be enjoyable. If it's not, then why eat something?

Another food item that can turn my stomach is dips that have already been dipped into. I do love taco dips, cheese dips, etc., when they're fresh and new. However, once people have started dipping into it, I can't help thinking about all the germs introduced by "double-dipping". A study has shown that dipping a half-eaten chip can transfer as many as 10,000 bacteria into the dip[7]. So I'll just pass on the chips and dip and save myself a few hundred calories.

Don't be afraid to waste food. I'm sure the mothers out

there may be horrified when I tell you it's okay to leave food on your plate. The truth is it really doesn't make any difference to the starving children in third-world countries if you eat the food or throw it away. Either way, the food is disposed of and can't be used by anyone else, but at least if you don't overeat, you'll be able to maintain a healthy weight and feel good about yourself. And by all means, donate to your favorite charity to help those kids in a way that may actually do some good!

Top 10 Charities

1. American Red Cross
2. Stop Hunger Now
3. Project Concern International
4. Children's Hunger Fund
5. Food for All
6. Children of the Americas
7. Africare
8. Heifer Project International
9. CARE
10. UNICEF

Sixty-nine percent of Americans usually eat everything or almost everything on their plates, according to a 2001 survey by the American Institute for Cancer Research[8]. You can choose to not be one of them. If you really don't want to waste food then you should try to not put as much on your plate in the first place. This is something we tend to learn as children. A young child doesn't know how to estimate how much he or she can actually eat, so parents will serve their food and determine the appropriate portion sizes for them. As the kids get older, we need to teach them how to recognize for themselves the correct portion size.

When you're eating out at a restaurant, set half of your meal aside for a doggie bag. Do this as soon as the meal is served, when you are able to accurately gauge how much half really amounts to. When eating at parties or family holidays, don't even put food on your plate that you know you shouldn't eat. If Grandma or some other well-meaning relative serves you, you'll just have to leave the excess amount on your plate and hope you're not offending the cook.

I like to eat only the best parts and leave the rest. For example, if I'm eating a sandwich, I usually leave the crust. The sandwich filling seems to run out before the bread does, so I just skip that leftover bread. Even Elvis uses this strategy. Sometimes when he eats a Danish or jelly doughnut, he'll eat the fruity middle first, and then leave the rest on his plate. When he eats burritos, he will leave the rolled up ends of the tortilla that don't have any more filling inside. This saves a few calories.

Don't go overboard on weekends. Researchers have found that the average person consumes an extra 115 calories per day on Fridays, Saturdays, and Sundays compared to the rest of the week[9]. That adds up to 350 calories each weekend, or 18,200 extra calories per year. Believe it or not, that could translate into a five-pound annual weight gain.

Try to maintain your good habits throughout the whole week. Two days of binge eating can not only undo the progress you've made, but can cause your weight to jump up even higher so that stricter measures will be required to bring it back under control. This can turn into yo-yo dieting, which has been shown to wreck your metabolism and lead to weight gain.

To avoid overeating on weekends, look for ways to combine family time with exercise, both indoors and out. You can go for a bike ride with your kids or spouse or play a pickup football game. Maybe you can work out at your local recreation center while the children enjoy playing basketball. In addition to getting some exercise, you'll be setting a good example for your kids.

If you enjoy cooking on the weekends, use the extra time to try out some healthy new recipes. You can also experiment with your old favorites and try to adapt them into healthier versions. Try new foods that you don't usually have time for on a busy weekday.

Limit dining out to just one meal per weekend. For me, that's always Friday night. However, if something comes up that you didn't plan for, such as a party or family get-together, try to compensate for the extra calories by planning extra physical activity, or eating less at another meal.

Analyze your food craving. Before reaching for that cookie or bag of potato chips, stop for a moment and think about your desire for the food. Are you really hungry or are you just looking for something to do? Are you eating out of habit or because you're actually hungry? If your hunger truly is a need for food, you'll have physical symptoms, too. You may feel light-headed or have a growling stomach. If your hunger is psychological, you'll feel more of an urge to eat something that looks good—such as a piece of chocolate cake. If you have physical hunger, have a healthy meal or snack. If the hunger seems psychological, distract yourself by taking a walk or calling a friend. Often you'll forget your "need" for food.

Now let's test your food knowledge by taking the fun quiz below.

1. If you lose weight through dieting without exercising, how much of the weight loss is from muscle?
    a)   10%
    b)   15%
    c)   25%

2. Which has more calories?
    a)   1/2 cup of pineapple
    b)   1/2 cup of coconut
    c)   1/2 cup of avocado

3. How much fat can a food contain when the label says 0 grams per serving?
    a)   up to half a gram
    b)   0 grams
    c)   3/4 gram

4. Which has more calories?
    a)   1/4 pound of shrimp

b)   1/4 pound meatloaf slice
c)   1/4 pound pork chop

5. Which container would a half-cup of cooked pasta most closely fit into?
a)   cupcake baking cup
b)   cereal bowl
c)   shot glass

6. Two tablespoons of butter could make a ball about the size of…
a)   a chickpea
b)   a golf ball
c)   a baseball

7. Which of the following condiments has less than 50 calories per serving?
a)   ketchup
b)   mustard
c)   pickle relish

8. How long would you have to walk to make up for eating a doughnut?
a)   15 minutes
b)   45 minutes
c)   two hours

Answers:

1.   c) 25%. It's very important to exercise when you're dieting to prevent your body from digesting your own muscles.

2.   b) coconut. A half cup of coconut has 142 calories, compared to avocado at 121 calories, and pineapple at only 38. Use coconut sparingly in recipes.

3.   a) up to half a gram – it's rounded down. So be careful when you read labels; the fat grams can add up, especially if you have more than one serving.

4.   c) pork chop (305 calories). Shrimp, at 173 calories per 1/4 pound serving, is a low calorie choice that is also high in protein and is a good source of healthy omega-3 acids. A serving of meatloaf has 241 calories.

5.   a) cupcake baking cup. A half-cup is considered a standard serving size of pasta. Think about how many servings are in a restaurant portion!

6.   b) a golf ball. Don't underestimate how much of this high-calorie (204), high-fat (23 grams) food you consume.

7.   All answers are correct. Use these condiments on burgers and sandwiches instead of higher calorie choices such as barbecue sauce or mayonnaise.

8.   b) 45 minutes. A glazed doughnut has about 230 calories, which would take about 45 minutes of brisk walking to burn off. You decide if it's worth it!

Your homework assignment

1. Select a few of the general eating strategies and enter them in Section 6 of your custom plan.
2. Continue gradually trying out the suggestions that appeal to you until you have hit on the combination that is most effective.

Part Four

Energize with Exercise

Chapter 8

Exercise Tips—the Basics

Let's face it: you can't really maintain a healthy weight unless you exercise. There's just no way around it—you know you have to do it. Maybe some of you really enjoy working out. However, I'm afraid most people think of it as a chore. How can you make exercise more interesting or fun? How can you sneak exercise into your daily routine so it's not extra effort? How can you get the most benefit in the shortest amount of time?

These are the questions I had, because I knew I could never stick to a boring routine. I tried exercise bikes, treadmills, and jogging and rarely stuck with any of them for more than 10 or 15 minutes at a time. Step aerobics classes and exercise tapes with dance music were slightly better, but still got tiresome after a while.

I finally came up with a routine that works for me and actually takes very little time. On four mornings each week, I do sit-ups, push-ups, and a few special exercises that target the abdominal muscles (my problem area). Twice a week, I lift free weights. Three times each week, I do a 30-minute circuit workout at a gym on my way home from work. In addition, I try to add unscheduled exercise such as going for a walk or a bicycle ride. I also try to burn calories throughout each day by just being active.

There are numerous health benefits associated with regular exercise. According to the U.S. Surgeon General, regular exercise effectively:

- Helps prevent heart disease and strokes
- Reduces the risk of developing diabetes
- Reduces the risk of developing high blood pressure (and also helps to reduce blood pressure in people for whom it is already high)
- Reduces the risk of developing colon cancer
- Fights depression and promotes improved stress management
- Builds and maintains healthy bones, muscles, and joints
- Helps older adults become stronger and better able to move about without falling
- Helps prevent back pain
- Helps prevent osteoporosis

Another important advantage of exercising is that it literally extends your life. A daily workout can add up to four years to your life, and just walking for 30 minutes a day can add as much as a year and a half[1].

Keeping all these benefits in mind, I'm sure you can understand why exercise is so important. This chapter contains basic exercise information that can help you decide which types of exercise are important to you. The next chapter offers suggestions on specific ways to add exercise and increased activity to your life.

Try weight training. Weight training, or strength training, will develop the strength and size of your skeletal muscles. It uses the force of gravity (in the form of weighted bars or dumbbells) to oppose the force generated by your muscles contracting. It requires the use of either free weights or a weight-training machine. You can use either dumbbells or kettlebells for free weights. I prefer dumbbells because I think they are easier to grip and balance.

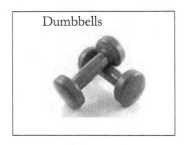

Dumbbells

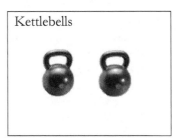

Kettlebells

Free weights, unlike weight machines, do not force you to use specific, controlled movements, and therefore they require more effort from your stabilizer, or core, muscles. This means free weight exercises can help you expend more energy in the same amount of time. You will be working on your core muscles at the same time as your arm or shoulder muscles.

Weight machines help prevent you from using poor form, so they are somewhat safer than free weights, especially for novices. Since you won't need to concentrate so much on maintaining good form, you can focus more on the effort you are putting into the exercise.

There are advantages to either approach. It's a matter of personal preference. Try both methods and see which works best for you.

In strength training, you will progressively increase the load on your muscles through incremental increases in weight or resistance. This is called overloading. The more you do, the more your body is capable of doing. You should increase your workload to avoid reaching a plateau. Do this by increasing the amount of weight lifted, changing the number of sets or repetitions, changing the exercises, or changing the type of resistance.

Sets with fewer reps can be performed with heavier weights if your goal is to build endurance. High weight/low repetition exercises are useful in maintaining or increasing the body's muscle mass, especially while dieting. This helps to prevent the metabolic slowdown that can lead to plateaus when dieting and can cause post-diet weight gain.

Sets with more repetitions but lighter weights will help

build strength and lean muscle, which will increase your metabolic rate so that you burn more calories, even when your body is at rest.

There is a trade-off between using more weight versus performing more repetitions. Generally, a heavier weight will increase your strength, while more repetitions will increase your muscle size or tone. Women don't need to worry about their muscles getting too large, though. That won't happen unless you're taking testosterone supplements. It's the testosterone in men that enables them to bulk up their muscles.

Weight lifting is especially important for people over 50. Many symptoms of aging are actually related to inactivity. Strength training can delay or even reverse loss of muscle mass and bone density in older people. It even helps improve your balance. Weight training can provide increased tendon and ligament strength, more flexibility, and improved muscle tone. It can also reduce the potential for injury, improve cardiac function, and elevate good cholesterol levels.

It's interesting to note that a pound of muscle is more compact than a pound of fat. This means that as you build body muscle, your clothes will fit better and you will lose inches, even if your weight stays the same.

Rest days are just as important as workout days. During these rest periods your muscles grow and change, so make sure you're not working the same muscle groups two days in a row.

> "For every hour you exercise, you get two hours of your life back." Jeff Galloway, author of "Running Until You're 100"

Remember to always warm up before you start lifting weights to help get your muscles warm and prevent injury. One way to warm up is to do some light cardio exercises such as a few jumping jacks. You could instead do a light set of each exercise before moving on to heavier weights.

Now this may seem hard, but you do need to lift and

lower your weights slowly. Don't use momentum to lift the weight. If you have to swing your arms or legs to get the weight up, it's probably too heavy for you.

To determine how much weight to lift, start with a light weight and lift it ten times. Rest for one or two minutes, and then perform a second set of ten consecutive lifts. If you can't do two sets of ten repetitions, switch to a lighter weight. If it seems too easy, switch to a heavier weight. You should be lifting enough weight so that you can just barely complete the last repetition. Once you are able to regularly do two or three sets, add more weight to the dumbbell or use a heavier weight. You should be able to increase the weight every two weeks or so.

I own various sizes of dumbbells, including 3-pound, 5-pound, 8-pound, and 10-pound weights. I keep them handy in the family room so I can pick them up whenever it's convenient for me. A great time for me to do my weights routine is when Elvis and I are watching a movie. While he's enjoying a bowl of ice cream in his recliner, I'll pick up the dumbbells.

Through experimentation, I have identified a series of 11 different exercises to perform with my dumbbells that work my upper body muscles. I do two sets of ten for each of them. For the more difficult ones, I use my 8-pound weights, but for the easier ones, I use 10-pound weights. Several years ago, when I was just starting to experiment with free weights, I used the lighter ones—3 and 5 pounds. I was able to gradually work up to the heavier weights. At this point, I plan to stick with my current level. I don't feel I need to increase the weight any more since I'm in maintenance mode now.

Find aerobic exercises that you enjoy. Aerobic refers to exercise that helps you use oxygen more efficiently by reaching and maintaining your target heart range—the safest range of heart beats per minute during exercise. You can calculate your target heart range by subtracting your age from 220 for women or from 226 for men. Then multiply your answer by 60% and by 80%. The lower number is the minimum rate needed to burn extra calories, while the higher number would be your upper goal as your fitness level improves.

For example, if you are a 55-year-old woman, subtract your age from 220 to arrive at 165. Multiplying this number by 60% gives you a lower range of 99 heart beats per minute, with an upper goal of 132 beats per minute (80% of 165). An easy way to find your heart rate is to count the beats for ten seconds, then multiply the result by 6. Alternatively, you could count your heartbeats for a full minute, but by then, your heart rate will probably have slowed down and the count may be less accurate.

Aerobic exercise is primarily intended to burn calories, increase endurance, and improve overall fitness, rather than strengthening specific muscles. Aerobic activities help make your heart stronger and more efficient. During the early part of exercise, your body uses stored carbohydrates for energy. As you continue exercising, you increase your heart rate and your body starts to use fat stores for energy.

Aerobic exercise has many of the same benefits as strength training but also has some additional ones. Here's a partial list:

- Improves bone calcium
- Improves high density ("good") cholesterol in the blood
- Improves handling of excess body heat
- Increases hemoglobin levels to help prevent anemia
- Improves resistance to cold
- Provides an emotional lift by increasing the body's production of endorphins
- Helps relax tense muscles, thereby relieving your body's stress response

There are many types of aerobic exercise. Running or jogging is basic, but has the big advantage of requiring very little equipment (just comfortable clothing and good running shoes). You can do it almost anywhere. Jogging around your neighborhood is convenient and familiar, or you could go to a local high school and use their running track.

Riding a bicycle is almost as convenient as running. I love

to hop on my bike in the summertime and ride around the neighborhood for about 20 minutes. We have several hills in the area, which provide a challenging workout that really gets my heart rate up.

I have recently taken up roller-blading. Don't say you're too old for it—if I can do it, you can too! I bought some inexpensive inline skates and plenty of pads for protection, and then headed to a local park. I may have gotten a few odd looks as I awkwardly tried to teach myself how to balance, but most people had a friendly smile for me. I felt that they respected my intentions, if not my form.

Dancing is another fun way to get in your aerobic exercise. Several of my friends who are in their fifties take tap-dancing lessons and really enjoy it. You can try swing dancing, square dancing, ballroom dancing—whatever appeals to you. Take a dance class with a partner and you'll have lots of fun while getting your exercise in.

The actual amount of calories burned while exercising will vary between individuals, depending on your weight. The heavier you are, the more calories it takes to perform an activity. The table below lists how many calories you can burn through various aerobic activities. As you can see, there are many ways to get in your regular exercise.

Table 8.1 - Calories burned through different activities

Activity - 1 hour	Weight 105-121 lbs	Weight 122-148 lbs	Weight 149-175 lbs	Weight 176-210 lbs
Aerobic dancing	348	396	468	516
Basketball	588	672	792	870
Bicycling	330	378	468	870
Bowling	223	253	299	333
Cleaning the house	465	529	623	694
Climbing stairs	354	402	474	528
Fast skating	486	558	654	720
Golf	198	228	264	294
Hiking (with backpack)	354	402	474	528
Jogging at 5 mph	516	552	690	762
Laundry	82	94	110	123
Mowing the lawn	210	240	288	312
Rock & roll dancing	198	228	264	294
Running at 8 mph	624	714	852	1038
Sexual activity	234	258	336	354
Shopping	175	198	234	260
Shoveling snow	474	546	648	750
Skiing - cross country	786	900	1068	1164
Skiing - downhill	468	624	738	798
Stationary bike at 10 mph	330	378	468	498
Stationary bike at 20 mph	702	798	936	1068
Swimming at 20 yds/min	234	270	318	408
Tennis	468	534	630	696
Walking at 2 mph	144	168	198	216
Walking at 4 mph	270	312	366	408
Watching TV	125	144	169	188
Yard work	301	341	403	448

Save time with circuit training. In circuit or interval training, strength exercises are alternated with endurance/aerobic exercises, thus combining the benefits of both a cardiovascular and a strength-training workout. A circuit refers to a group of activities or stations positioned around the facility that are to be visited in sequence. Each strength-training station has some type of resistance equipment, such as a hydraulic weight machine or free weights, with alternating aerobic spaces for doing jumping jacks, jogging in place, or other aerobic activities to keep your heart rate up. When performing a circuit, you complete the activity at one station before you proceed to the next station. Then you continue until you have passed through all stations once or twice (as required) or until a certain time requirement has been met, such as 30 minutes. You will usually work each station for a very short period of time—30 or 60 seconds.

Many women's fitness centers are based on interval training, but you can also set up your own circuit at home by alternating 30 seconds of free weights with 30 seconds of the treadmill or stationary bike. The variety keeps it from getting dull, plus you can efficiently burn calories and build strength within the same 30-minute period.

> "Exercise has been proven to lower the lifetime risk of getting breast cancer.[2]"

Studies show circuit training especially helps women to achieve their goals and maintain them longer than other forms of exercise or diet[3]. Because it is not geared towards bulking up, women tend to lose weight more quickly with circuit workouts.

Add calisthenics to your routine. The word calisthenics is derived from a combination of Greek words meaning "beautiful strength". Sounds motivating, doesn't it? I'm sure we all want to feel both beautiful and strong. Here are some descriptions of basic types of calisthenics exercises.

Sit-ups or crunches: Start with your back on the floor, knees bent, and bottoms of your feet against the floor. Lift your shoulders off the floor by tightening the abdominal muscles and bringing your chest closer to your knees. Then lower your back to the floor with a smooth movement. This trains your abdominal muscles.

> "Older women who exercise are three times less likely to catch a cold as those who don't work out[4]."

For many years I did 50 sit-ups as part of my morning routine. I have to admit they were my least favorite exercise. In an attempt to add more variety, I purchased an abdominal roller gadget to replace the sit-ups. I now do 15 repetitions of the ab roller. It takes a lot less time than doing 50 sit-ups, but I feel it is just as effective.

Push-ups: Start face down on the floor, palms against the floor under your shoulders, with your toes curled up against the floor. Push your body up with your arms while keeping your body in a straight line from head to toe. Lower your body to within a few inches of the floor and repeat. Don't rest on the floor when you descend. This exercise works your chest, shoulder, and tricep muscles. (In Great Britain, push-ups are called press-ups. I'm sure using this term will impress all your friends.)

You can start out by doing push-ups on your knees instead of your toes. These are referred to as "girly" push-ups (as least that's how Elvis refers to them.) Once you have strengthened your arms and shoulders enough, you can gradually work up to "manly" push-ups. Men's push-ups are definitely more difficult for women to do. Not only do we have less upper body strength than men, we also have a lower center of gravity. For many years I did girly push-ups each morning, until one day Elvis challenged me to try doing the standard version. At first I could barely do one, but I kept at it until I reached the point where I could do 25. That's now part of my routine, four times each week.

Another variation on the basic push-up is the tap push-up. To perform this version, do a normal push-up, but when you are in the raised position, lift one hand from the floor and tap the opposite wrist. This type of push-up is somewhat easier as it gives you a chance to catch your breath between repetitions.

> "Exercising 90 minutes per week saves an average of $2,200 per year in healthcare costs[5]."

Pull-ups: Start by grabbing an overhead bar using an overhand (palms facing away from you) grip. Pull yourself up to chin level with the bar in front of your head, then return to the starting position in a slow, controlled manner. Avoid making jerky movements to gain leverage. This exercise primarily trains your upper back muscles and the forearms. You can also use an underhand grip variation (called a chin-up) to work both the back and biceps. I find this method to be somewhat easier for me.

It never occurred to me to even try doing pull-ups as part of my routine until one time when Elvis and I were taking a walk during a vacation. We came across a chin-up bar that was part of a walking circuit. Just for fun, we tried to see if either of us could do a pull-up. Elvis managed to do one, and I surprised myself by doing two (barely). After that, I wanted to continue working on it, since it's one of the few physical things I can do better than him. For my last birthday, Elvis gave me my own personal chin-up bar and installed it in our basement so I can do them any time I feel like it.

Doing pull-ups or chin-ups may seem too strenuous to most women. I must admit it took me a long time to be able to do more than one or two. I usually do only four or five of them at a time, four or five times a week. Even though they are very difficult, it's important for women to do exercises like pull-ups that help develop our upper body strength. That tends to be a weakness for most of us. Also, having a more muscular upper body gives your body better overall proportions and can help balance out a pear-shaped body.

Squats: Stand with your feet shoulder-width apart. Squat down as far as possible, bringing your arms forward parallel to the floor. Return to a standing position and repeat. If this basic squat isn't challenging enough for you, try a variation. One method is lifting one leg off the floor in front of you, putting both arms in front of you for balance, and then squatting. This is called a one-legged squat or pistol. Love that name. Another variation is to hold 5-pound weights in each hand with arms down while squatting.

Squats are great for working the quadriceps, hamstrings, calves, and gluteals. This is possibly the best exercise there is for developing a shapely bottom.

Calf-raises: Stand on a step or platform with an edge where you can let your heels hang. Use your heels to lift your body on the balls of your feet, then slowly return to the starting position. This exercise works your upper calf muscles on your lower legs. You can do the same movements in a seated position to work the lower calf muscles. This exercise can prevent the dreaded "cankles", where your calf and ankle seem to blend together.

Your homework assignment:

1. Choose which of the exercise strategies above you are willing to try out. Don't feel you need to make a long-term commitment to each idea at this time. Try to give it three - six weeks, however, to really determine if it is something that is effective for you and is something you are willing to stick with. Write these items down in Section 7 of your plan.
2. Identify any problem areas of your body that you really want to tone up. List those, too, along with specific exercises that will help improve your target areas.

Chapter 9

Everyday Exercise Strategies

It's important to not only exercise regularly, but also to be active throughout each day. Having an active versus a sedentary lifestyle will burn extra calories and keep your metabolism revved up. Inactivity has been shown to contribute to aging-related diseases, such as cardiovascular disease, diabetes, and osteoporosis[1]. It can also affect the aging process itself and reduce life expectancy. Regular exercise is actually anti-aging—another great reason to stay active. Exercise also increases blood flow to ligaments, muscles, and joints, which strengthens the core muscles that support your spine.

This chapter will provide you with lots of ideas on how to incorporate additional physical activity into your routine. Some of them may sound familiar and others may be a little more creative. As you read, think about which ones can fit easily into your personal lifestyle and habits. You can probably guess that I'll ask you to add them to your plan at the end of the chapter. You guessed right!

Go for a walk. The many advantages of walking include its low cost, convenience, low impact, safety, and of course, effectiveness. Most people are able to walk, even if they're not ready for more strenuous activities. You don't need any special equipment and you can do it almost anywhere. I love taking walks around my neighborhood in good weather. In poor weather, the mall or civic center are good alternatives.

Walking is most effective when done at a brisk pace, at least four miles per hour. You can actually double the number of calories burned by walking on a soft surface, such as sand (my personal favorite) or uneven grass. You can also increase the intensity by using hand weights as you walk. You might want to try wearing ankle weights or a weight vest to burn even more calories.

If you decide to walk for exercise, tailor a plan that will work for you so you'll be able to stick with it. Decide what time of day works best for your schedule (and motivation). Plan in advance where you will walk and whom you will walk with.

Target your own problem areas. Decide which parts of your body you really want to focus on. Don't waste your limited, valuable time working on areas that don't really need it. Sometimes you just need to pick your battles. After all, there are over 600 muscles in your body and you can't possibly exercise all of them in your workouts.

In my case, I always try to do exercises that tone the stomach and lower abdomen because these are problem areas for me. However, I don't bother with lunges because I feel my legs and rear end are fine. I love to try new routines targeting the abdominal muscles. Many magazines offer innovative techniques, such as butt lifts (lie on your back with your legs straight up in the air, then try to raise up and hold for a few seconds) or leg scissors (lie on your back with legs in the air, scissor them out while lifting arms and shoulders off the floor). I've also found a variety of exercises in the health section of the newspaper. When the same old routine gets stale, I try out some new ones I have found and clipped out.

You may choose a different area to work on. The idea is to use your time wisely and don't get burned out by trying to exercise too much.

Plan ahead for your workouts. In general, most Americans are pressed for time. This may be especially true for women, with the multiple demands placed on our time from family, work, friends, and volunteer activities. In order to squeeze exercise into our crowded schedules, we need to plan for it. The more specific your plan, the more successful you will be in achieving it. Don't say, "I'm going to exercise this week." Instead, say "I'm going to spend 30 minutes on the treadmill on Tuesday at 4:30" or "I will go to the fitness center right after work on Monday, Wednesday, and Friday."

It's even better if you write down your exercise plans. It might seem a little obsessive, but try to put together a plan for the whole week on Sunday evening. This gives you concrete goals and structure so that the week doesn't get away from you. Otherwise, you may suddenly realize on Saturday that you haven't found the time to work out at all. This can leave you feeling out of control and frustrated.

Mornings are a great time to exercise because you can "get it out of the way" so you're not tempted to find excuses later for not following through. It will also help rev up your metabolism for the rest of the day.

If you're not a morning person, consider exercising during your lunch hour or in the evening. Experts say afternoon workouts are actually more productive. Your blood pressure is lower, your muscles are warmer, and your breathing capacity is larger in the late afternoon.

The important thing is to exercise when you can. Although the experts generally recommend against working out late in the evening, it does work for some people. An example is Janice V., who lost 60 pounds by working out to exercise tapes at night before bedtime. She never had trouble getting to sleep and it was the only time of the day that she was able to fit in her exercise. Sometimes you have to trust your own judgment and experience instead of believing everything the experts tell you.

Try organized exercise. Many people prefer some structure to their exercise. For them, organized activities and programs may work best. I really enjoy working out at a ladies-only club that offers circuit training. They provide the equipment and the routine, but I am able to go at whatever time is convenient for me, usually on my way home from work.

You may prefer to attend exercise classes, such as step aerobics or spinning. You may even want to hire a personal trainer. You can sign up for a martial arts class, indoor tennis, rock climbing, horseback riding, or volleyball. Use your imagination and I'm sure you'll come up with a program that's right for you.

Exercise alone. Louise V. was determined to get into shape and lose weight. She tried working out at gyms. She tried aerobics classes. But she found that whenever she worked out with or around other people, she felt de-motivated. She compared herself to the people she saw who she perceived to be slimmer, in better shape, and more proficient at using the machines or doing the exercises.

So Louise tried working out at home alone, using exercise tapes to follow along with. This resulted in a higher level of personal motivation as she pushed herself to work harder and harder. Working out on her own eliminated the discouraging feeling she got around others and helped her reach her goal.

Choosing to exercise alone also gives you a little more flexibility, which can be critical if you have a very busy schedule. You may not have two hours to spare to drive to a gym and work out, but you may be able to squeeze in at least 30 minutes of exercise right at home, either by using your own exercise equipment such as a treadmill or stationary bicycle, or by simply working out with weights or to an exercise DVD.

Work out with someone you care about. Working out with your spouse or good friend can really keep you motivated and make the time pass more pleasantly. A recent study found that 94% of spouses who worked out together stuck to their exercise plans, compared with only 57% of those who went at it alone[2].

I used to do my circuit workouts with my daughter, Vicki, when we both lived in the same city. We met at the fitness center after work and squeezed in a mother-daughter visit while exercising. Working out together kept us both motivated to show up each day and gave us an opportunity to catch up on each other's news.

If you have an exercise buddy, you'll be much more likely to stay with your plan. Your buddy can provide encouragement at times when you may not be enthusiastic about working out, and you can provide the same support for your buddy.

> "Lack of exercise may cause your DNA to age faster[3]."

Exercise for a bigger cause than yourself. Try signing up for a charity walk/run, like the MS Bike Tour (www.nationalmssociety.org), which raises funds for multiple sclerosis research, or Race for the Cure (www.komen.org/race), which benefits breast cancer research. You'll help yourself stay fit while also helping others. Plus, after hitting up friends and family for donations, you'll be motivated to reach your goal to avoid the embarrassment of not following through. In the weeks and months leading up to your race, you'll need to stay (or get) in shape, so that will keep you going to the gym.

Alternate your weights routine. One way to spice up your exercise routine is to vary your weights and repetitions. Use heavier weights with fewer reps for a while (several weeks) then switch to lighter weights with more reps. This keeps it fresh and also gives your muscles a bit of a change. The lighter weights are easier, but the heavier weights take less time, so each has an advantage over the other.

You can motivate yourself to stick with it by focusing on the advantage of the approach you're currently using. Tell yourself, "This isn't so tough, I only need to do 8 reps" or "I can easily handle this, it's only 5 pounds."

Build activity into daily habits. This is one of my favorite tricks. In addition to performing "real" exercise, being physically active will burn off calories and keep your metabolism revving. Try to never be completely still. Work in some type of jiggling or fidgeting when you're working at your desk, standing in a line, or watching television. Bounce up and down on the balls of your feet while brushing your teeth. Tap your feet to the music while driving. March in the shower as you wash your hair. It may sound silly, but all of this movement adds up throughout the course of a day. In fact, according to scientific studies, you can burn up to 350 calories a day just by fidgeting[4]. Even just standing burns about 50% more calories than sitting.

Think of ways you can be more active in your daily life. Jog your dog instead of just walking him. Every time you shop at the mall, first walk briskly around the mall twice before you start shopping. You can do this in any kind of weather. When you go to work, park a long distance from the entrance so you'll be forced to walk further. Better yet, ride a bike to work if possible. Think of all the gas you'll save too!

See the list below for a few more ideas for building activity into your regular routine. Then see if you can come up with your own ideas for getting some automatic exercise.

Top 10 Ways to Get Exercise in your Daily Routine

1.   Park in the first spot you see, no matter how far from the entrance.
2.   Take the stairs instead of the escalator/elevator.
3.   Tap your feet while sitting at stoplights.
4.   Do squats while you brush your teeth.
5.   Carry your groceries to your car instead of using the cart (if it's a small enough load).
6.   Walk over to your coworker's desk instead of calling them.
7.   If it's a nice day and you're going somewhere close by, walk or bike instead of driving.
8.   Lift hand weights during commercials while watching TV.
9.   Pace when you're talking on the telephone.
10.   Use gestures—talk with your hands and your body.

Find creative ways to add exercise. Even the little things can add up when it comes to burning calories. Sometimes you may find yourself being inactive out of habit when you could actually be doing something. As an example, a group of my friends and I take turns hosting quarterly dinner parties. After enjoying a nice meal, many times we will move to the family room and play some party games, such as Pictionary or Trivial Pursuit. While most of the group is content to sit in comfortable chairs and relax, I volunteer to get up to distribute the pencils and paper or pass the dice around. Someone has to do it, and it allows me the opportunity to move around instead of just sitting still.

Another example is when I play ping-pong with Elvis or the kids. Since we are not exactly expert players, the ball often flies out of control and ends up on the other side of the room. I am usually the person who retrieves the balls. When we play tennis, I get even more exercise chasing stray balls. I don't look at it as an interruption to the game, though. I just think of it as part of the fun and an easy way to build in more activity.

I live in a two-story house so I try to get the maximum benefit out of going up and down stairs. When I'm heading up the steps, I jog instead of walking. It's become such a habit that I don't even think about it any more.

If you live in a two-story house or a ranch house with a basement, you can use your stairs for built-in exercise. Don't focus on being efficient. Instead, take two trips instead of one. When I'm carrying clean clothes from the laundry room on the main floor to the bedrooms upstairs, I'll make one trip with Elvis's clothes and a second trip with my own things. That gives me twice the exercise.

Another trick is to maximize the benefits of your weight training by doing something aerobic during the 30 seconds between sets. I will do a set of exercises using my free weights, then march around the room for 30 seconds before starting the next set. It doesn't take any longer to do the workout and it burns a few extra calories while also keeping my heart rate up.

Make the treadmill exciting. Using a treadmill to get your exercise has many advantages. If you have the equipment at home, you can choose to use it at your convenience, whenever you can work it in to your schedule. Be sure to keep it ready to use. Don't use it for hanging laundry!

> "Moderate exercise boosts the immune system to fight infections more easily.[5]"

However, a treadmill can get boring if you do the same routine every time. To keep it more interesting, try alternating faster intervals with less vigorous intervals, or adding an incline. The fast periods and inclines will burn more calories, build stronger leg muscles, and improve your heart health. You also might be able to sign up for a treadmill class. These classes add energizing music along with an instructor leading you through combinations of walking and jogging to keep things interesting.

If you work out at a gym on a treadmill, you can do it side-by-side with a buddy and catch up on your socializing while you're walking. That's a great way to make the time fly.

Obvious ways to avoid boredom during a treadmill workout are to watch a television program, listen to music or a book on tape, or chat with a friend on a hands-free telephone. Take advantage of your multi-tasking skills to do two things at once.

One more suggestion for keeping your treadmill workout interesting is to set it up near a picture window. Looking at nature can be soothing and calming. Researchers have found that viewing rural scenery while running on a treadmill produces substantial reductions in blood pressure[6]. Once when I was on a Caribbean cruise, I used the treadmill in the ship's fitness center. It was positioned in front of a huge window facing the front of the ship. As I jogged, I could see the beautiful ocean all around me. It was easy to get lost in the gorgeous tropical atmosphere and lose all track of time.

Work out to music. I love music, especially good old rock 'n roll. I find music to be very energizing. If you work out to music, you'll find the time goes by faster and more pleasantly. In fact, a recent study found that people who exercised to music were able to work out an average of 11% longer than those who worked out in either a noisy environment or in silence[7]. Pick your favorite iPod playlist or tune in to your favorite radio station and you'll have fun while you get in your exercise.

Create an exercise budget. How about budgeting for your exercise? Itemize each type of exercise you are planning to do and assign a number of units to each. For example, a 30-minute circuit workout could be five points, going for a brisk 20-minute walk could be four points, and doing 25 push-ups might be two points. Then set a goal of how many exercise units you want to accomplish each week. As you go through the week, log in the points you've earned until you reach your goal. Don't forget to include one-pointers, too. If you do enough of them, even if they are simple activities like going up a flight of stairs or taking your dog for a walk, they will add up to help you reach your weekly goal.

Another advantage of using this approach is that it keeps you honest and improves the accuracy of how much you exercise. Most exercisers, at least at first, are far too generous with their estimates of exercise intensity and time, amount of weight lifted, and the frequency of their workouts. Keeping an exercise log will help to prevent overestimating your activity level.

Wear a pedometer. A pedometer is a great motivator to get you to walk more. Whenever I wear a pedometer, I naturally start competing with myself to see how many steps I can get in for the day. Perhaps this explains why researchers have found that wearing a step counter leads to weight loss and lower blood pressure. In an 18-week study, people who used a pedometer walked an average of seven additional miles weekly and also lowered their body mass index by an average of 0.4 points[8].

Pedometers can be fancy, but you can also find inexpensive ones at your local discount store. I paid under $5.00 for mine. You should set a goal of walking 10,000 steps each day. Use the pedometer for a day to establish your normal baseline step count, then try adding 100 more steps each day until you reach the 10,000 level. If the weather doesn't allow for walking outdoors, consider an indoor track or treadmill.

Measure the right things to track your progress. Don't think your exercise plan isn't working if you're not losing weight each time you step on a scale. If you're building muscle and burning fat, your weight may stay the same or even go up slightly. You can measure your fitness progress in better ways. Some suggestions are:

- Track your heart rate after a certain level of exercise
- Measure the distance you can cover in a certain amount of time
- Track the amount of weight you can lift
- Test your blood pressure or cholesterol numbers periodically

You can then graph these numbers to see trends and progress (I know, I'm a geek, but I love charts).

Other ways to monitor progress might not involve specific measures, but could be more subjective. You may feel better physically, your clothes may fit more comfortably, or you may be able to do daily chores more easily. Writing down your progress in any of these areas can be a great motivator.

Focus on quality versus quantity. Many people go to the gym out of habit, put in some time, and then head back home without even breaking a sweat. They may think they are doing themselves some good, even if they are lifting weights so light that very little effort is required or if they are walking on a treadmill at a very leisurely pace. I've noticed some women at my fitness center who just seem to go through the motions with a minimum of exertion, with not a hair out of place. If you are one of these people, ask yourself, "Why am I exercising? What do I want to get out of this?"

Although any activity is better than doing nothing and these people are at least motivated enough to show up at the gym, they would get much better results if they focused on quality instead of quantity. You can still enjoy your workouts, but you need to get serious about what you are doing to increase the quality of every movement. When you are exercising with purpose and pushing both your aerobic capacity and your strength you will find you can get better results in half the time.

Vary your exercise routine. Not only does it get boring to do the same routine day after day, but your body also adapts to it by becoming very efficient at doing the same exercise over and over. This is great for building endurance or performance, but not so great for increasing your strength or maintaining weight loss. If you always do the same workout for the same amount of time you will eventually hit a plateau where you fail to see any additional results.

One way to overcome this plateau is to change your workouts every few weeks or months. You can change the type of exercise you do, the length of time you spend exercising, the amount of weight you lift, or the number of repetitions.

Another way to give yourself a break in your routine is to just allow yourself a day off from exercising. You can work hard during the week, and then relax a little on the weekends. You'll be rested and motivated when you resume your fitness program in the week ahead.

On the other hand, weekends might actually be a good time to get your workouts in since you may have a little more free time. It's a good idea to get it out of the way early by planning your exercise for Saturday morning before you slip into that weekend relaxation mode. Try something different for the weekends to spice up your workouts. If you normally do a circuit workout during the week, maybe you can jog or take a spinning class on a Saturday or Sunday to add a little variety.

Elle Marie

Your homework assignment:

1. Choose which of the exercise tips above you are willing to try out. Write these items down in Section 7 of your plan.
2. Now try to think of any other ways you can add more activity to your daily routine. Enter them into your custom plan.

Part Five

Putting It All Together

Chapter 10

Tips & Tricks

In this chapter, I'll give you some real-life strategies for resisting temptation, shaving calories from your daily food intake, working exercise into your daily routine, and staying motivated. Some tips may seem a little unusual, or even unorthodox, but try to keep an open mind. I prefer to think of them as creative tricks. Remember, real people have successfully used these methods to stay in control of their fitness and weight.

Make a calorie budget. Treat your eating like money. Budget your calories so that if you spend more on one thing, you must make up for it somewhere else. Think of each day as a pay period with a limited amount of calories available. You have to get through the rest of the day within your budget. Then the next day, you get "paid" again with a day's worth of calories to spend.

This approach can teach you to choose the foods you eat carefully. You don't want to use up your whole daily budget on one meal (which can happen if you have a fast food hamburger, fries, and a milkshake), because then you'll have to fast for the rest of the day.

Carry a purse-size calorie counter with you everywhere so you can easily determine whether a specific food will fit into your budget.

Be sure to get enough sleep. If you don't get enough sleep, your levels of cortisol (the so-called "stress hormone") will rise. This causes you to gain weight because your metabolism slows down and you're not burning calories efficiently. By getting an adequate amount of sleep each night, you're actually helping to stabilize your metabolism.

Don't take this tip to the extreme, though. A friend of mine told me that she was afraid lack of sleep was causing her to gain weight. So when she found herself with a little unexpected free time one afternoon, she debated whether to work out or just take a nap. She ended up choosing the nap, rationalizing it would help her lose weight. Call me crazy, but I'm pretty sure she would have burned a few more calories by choosing to exercise.

Create a reward system. Reward yourself for exercising or sticking to your eating plan. Put a dollar in a jar every time you work out or each day you don't go over your calorie allotment. Set a specific monetary goal, and when you reach it, treat yourself to a non-food shopping splurge. Or you might want to save the money for a special reward, such as a beach vacation where you can feel confident wearing your swimsuit.

If you respond better to shorter-term rewards, you can come up with other ways of treating yourself, such as taking 30 minutes to relax and read a novel or enjoy a bubble bath.

> *"Extra pounds increase the load on your spine, leading to disc degeneration.[1]"*

Decide what you are going to eat in advance. At the beginning of each day you can plan your meals and snacks for the entire day. This simplifies your decision-making because you've already decided what you are going to eat.

Use this advance planning technique when you eat out as well. Plan what you will order before you arrive at a restaurant.

Once you've made a decision, don't even look through the menu or you may change your mind and end up with a higher-calorie choice.

A woman at my fitness center came up with the unique approach of putting all of her food for the day in a cooler each morning. She could eat anything from the cooler any time she wanted, but once it was empty, that was all she got until the next day. It may not be practical for you to use an actual cooler and carry it around with you all day long, but you can still use the basic concept. Write down your meal plan and refer to it so you know what you can eat that day. Spread it out however you like throughout the day, but when the "cooler" is empty, no more eating!

Weigh in daily. I weigh myself each morning so I can see if I'm staying within my allowed 3-pound range. If my weight creeps up above the upper limit of my range, I count calories for a few days or a week until I am back in my comfort zone.

Once when I was in London on a business trip, I discovered the hotel had provided a bathroom scale in my room. I was very excited, because now I could continue my daily weigh-ins without a ten-day break! Unfortunately, the scale didn't use pounds for measuring (I guess because that would mean money over there) but instead some unknown (at least to me) British unit of weight. I wasn't sure if it was some kind of metric unit like kilograms or something else called a stone. However, I faithfully weighed myself each day, even though I wasn't sure what 8.3 meant or whether I was staying within my normal weight range. At least I could tell if I was up or down each day, and adjust my fish 'n chips intake accordingly. And 8.3 sure *sounded* good!

Daily weigh-ins really work for me, but they're not for everyone. If you're the type of person who gets upset over minor daily fluctuations, try weighing yourself only once a week. You don't want to lose confidence or motivation just because the number on the scale may be a little higher one day.

It's never too late or too little. Don't give up on yourself if you have a temporary setback. It's never too late to start eating right. Even if you're halfway through a bag of Oreos, you can stop and not eat the rest of the bag. Even if you eat a Big Mac, you can have a diet soda. That may seem inconsistent but you still can save hundreds of calories. I've seen people overeat because of the holidays, a special event, or some other excuse, and then they decide they'll never be able to eat healthy so they stop trying altogether. Change that attitude! You can decide to eat sensibly starting right now.

The same advice applies to exercising. Even elderly people who have never exercised in their lives can benefit from beginning workouts in their retirement years. It's never too late to build strength and endurance. In fact, the benefits to older people from even just a little regular exercise are noticeable. They can improve their balance and gain strength to help with everyday activities, such as getting out of chairs and washing dishes.

Try to focus on small, short-term goals. As you succeed in meeting these goals, your self-confidence will build. You'll know that you can stick to a plan. An example of a small goal is to look at one day at a time, or even one afternoon at a time.

"If I can't do this workout properly, then there is no point in working out." Do you ever have thoughts like this? Instead, tell yourself that even a five minute walk is better than five minutes on the couch or even ten minutes of light weights is better than nothing. This is especially important when exercising after recovering from a sickness or injury. You may feel like you took one step forward but fell three steps backward. Go easy on yourself. Don't give up! Something is better than nothing.

Know your weaknesses. If you know what your weaknesses and temptations are, you'll be able to compensate for them. Maybe you have cravings late at night. If so, you can compensate by allowing yourself a limited treat at night or by eating less earlier in the day. If sweets are your downfall, switch to sugar-free or low calorie versions of your favorite treats or limit your portions. Many foods now are available in 90 or 100-calorie packages, making it simple to control your portion size. Planning ahead will enable you to come up with ways to work around your weak spots.

Serve food directly onto your plate. It's much too tempting to take a second or even a third helping when you put serving bowls on the dinner table. The best plan is to immediately put any leftover food in storage bowls and put them away after you portion your plate so the sight of it does not tempt you.

Don't eat before you go out to parties. I know the diet experts tell you to have a healthy snack before you go out so you're not as hungry, but I have found that when I do, I tend to eat just as much at the party. Instead, I save a few calories by not having a pre-party meal. After all, I'm not really eating the party food because I'm hungry, but because it just looks too good to pass up!

Use exercise as an outlet. When you're stressed, upset, or even excited, exercise can be very calming. Suppose that on your way home from work, you've had a close call in rush hour traffic and nearly had an accident. Your adrenaline may be flowing fast. As soon as you walk in the door, head for the treadmill and exercise it out of your system.

I like to work out right after work. When I arrive at the gym, my head is full of things I need to do, people I need to call, and reports I need to write. But by the time I've worked out, I'm able to put those things at the back of my mind and I can head home in a much calmer state of mind.

Use exercise as a warm-up—literally. If you tend to get cold like me, you can use exercise to quickly warm you up. I'm usually cold when everyone else is comfortable, so I don't like to bother everyone by turning up the heat (or turning down the air-conditioning). Instead, I'll do a few sets with hand weights or a few push-ups. The exercise revs up my metabolism, burns off a few calories, and saves me the trouble of finding a sweater.

Brush your teeth. I got this tip from Lynn, a friend of mine.

One night she was contemplating having a little more wine with her dinner (since the bottle was almost empty and she didn't want to wrestle with the cork anyway) but then she decided to let someone else finish it. Just to be sure she didn't get tempted, Lynn decided to go brush her teeth. She knew it wouldn't be worth it to have another sip of wine if it meant she was going to have to go back and brush again.

If you get into the habit of brushing your teeth immediately after dinner (or after your planned-for snack), you may be able to avoid the temptation of eating something else. Brushing your teeth provides a mental signal to yourself that mealtime is over. This is also great for your dental health.

Enjoy dessert. Another way to trick yourself into eating less at a meal is to go ahead and have your dessert before you're completely full from dinner. Once you have that sweet taste in your mouth, you probably won't want to eat anything else. Dessert also acts as a signal that the meal is over, since it's usually the last thing you eat.

Philippe M., another friend of mine, uses this strategy to avoid second and third helpings. He has found that when he eats something sweet, it "kills the salty flavor" so then he isn't tempted to have another helping of dinner. This may not work for everyone, but if you're already going to have dessert anyway, it's best to go ahead and eat it so you can quit eating more calories at dinner.

Drink more liquids. You may really be thirsty, not hungry, when you think you are experiencing a hunger pang. Drink some coffee or tea and see if that does the trick. Water, diet soda, or light fruit juice can help fill you up until it's time to eat.

I like to drink lots of water with meals and snacks. I use a technique referred to as "sip—nibble—repeat". This tends to slow down the meal, making me feel like I'm actually eating more since it's taking longer. Many people I dine with will have eaten twice as much food as I have in the same amount of time. The water also helps to fill me up and make me feel satisfied.

Here's another great reason to drink a sip of water between each bite of food: You have taste receptors in your mouth that are sensitive to the taste of food. However, the second bite of the same food won't taste quite as good because of a phenomenon called sensory adaptation[2]. The sensitivity of the taste receptors decreases with more bites of the same food. However, if you drink water between bites, your receptors recover their sensitivity and the next bite will taste just as good as the first. So sipping water between bites actually makes your food taste better!

If you don't drink enough water, your body could get in the habit of storing water. This fluid retention equals extra unwanted weight. When you drink more water, you are actually teaching your body that it no longer needs to hoard water. You should drink at least 64 ounces of water (about eight glasses) a day to combat fluid retention. If you don't like plain water, try adding sliced lemons for a little flavor.

Drinking very cold water can actually burn calories[3]. Your body's normal temperature is approximately 98.6° Fahrenheit (or 37° Celsius), while ice water is about 40°F (0°C). When you consume ice water, your body has to bring its temperature up by almost 60°F (37°C). It takes .001 calories to raise the temperature of one gram of water by 1°C. That means that to raise the temperature of a 16-ounce (473 gram) glass of ice water by 60°F, your body would burn about 17.5 calories (473 times 37 times .001). Drinking 64 ounces (eight glasses) of water daily will burn 70 calories. This is an easy way to burn an additional 490 calories per week.

In addition, drinking lots of water will improve digestion, give you a clearer complexion, and act as a natural appetite suppressant. One more advantage of drinking lots of water is that it helps prevent dark circles under your eyes, which can be caused by dehydration.

Avoid food when you're under stress. It can be very tempting to overeat in response to stress. You may not even realize you are doing it if you are distracted and preoccupied with personal problems. However, trying to use food to cope with your stress will only add calories to your daily total and probably increase the stress level as you feel yourself losing control.

Stress releases a chemical reaction that actually triggers fat cells to grow and multiply in number. A recent animal study showed stress can cause weight gain even if total calorie intake remains the same[4].

Instead of eating, you could exercise, call a friend, take a walk, or go online to find a support group. Try to stay away from the kitchen and any other situations where you will be surrounded by food. Also keep in mind exercise lowers stress hormones, making it an even better alternative.

Wait it out. If you get a craving, try to wait ten minutes and see if you still want the food. It's possible you'll get busy and will just forget about it. You can also chew sugarless gum or drink coffee, tea, or water to tide you over until the next meal. A research study found chewing gum before an afternoon snack helped reduce hunger and diminish cravings[5]. People in the study reduced their calorie intake from snacks by an average of 25 calories. Even small changes in calories can have an impact in the long term.

Your homework assignment

1. Select any of the tips and tricks from this chapter and enter them in Section 8 of your custom plan.

Chapter 11

Living the Thin Life

I've told you a lot about myself and some of the strategies and tricks I use to eat healthy (without constantly dieting) and to include exercise in my life (without being a slave to the gym). Now I'd like to show you my own personal plan that puts it all together. Here's what it looks like:

*****

Elle's Personal Plan

Section 1 - My Motivators

I want to be strong and healthy
I want my husband to compliment me
I want to feel self-confident
I want all my clothes to fit me and look good on me

Section 2 - My Lame Excuses

It's natural for people to gain weight as they get older
I have better (more fun) things to do than exercise
I don't want to give up my favorite foods

Section 3 - I Can Resist Temptation

I will have only one bite of a special treat
I won't keep junk food in the house
I will chew sugarless gum to fend off my hunger until mealtime
I will remind myself of my motivators

Section 4 - My Ideal Weight

115 pounds (BMI 19.9)

Section 5 - I Am A ...

 deer

Section 6 - My Eating Strategies

Substitute lower calorie versions for my favorite foods
Use Splenda in coffee and recipes
Eat slowly
Eat soup for lunch on weekdays
Treat myself occasionally with a Dove chocolate

Section 7 - My Exercise Program

Perform a circuit workout 3 times a week
Do calisthenics every Monday, Wednesday, Friday, and Saturday
Do a free weights routine twice a week
Go roller-blading in the park once a week in the summer
Go for walks with my husband

Section 8 - My Personal Tips

Drink eight glasses of water each day
Weigh myself each day and write it down in a log
Never have second helpings

Each day that I follow my eating plan, I will enjoy a diet pudding after dinner

*****

You can see how I've picked the ideas that work for me personally and inserted them into each section of the plan. Now I have a handy guide that's easy to follow and that I know will be successful for me.

Next I'd like to tell you about some real people I know and how they each were able to create unique and successful plans to fit their own lifestyles.

Mary V. was athletic in high school and stayed in great shape throughout her twenties. After having three children, however, she began to slowly gain weight, adding a few pounds each year. Her life was very busy with all of her children's activities, including home schooling and sports, so taking care of herself became a low priority. After her two oldest children went away to college, she began working outside the home full-time and needed to shop for a new wardrobe since most of the clothes in her closet were baggy sweatshirts and jeans.

Mary found shopping discouraging and felt nothing looked good on her. That gave her the motivation she needed to lose some weight and get back in shape. Her strategy was to give up all sweets—cold turkey. Since the day she made that decision, she has not eaten one dessert or sweet snack. This was effective for her because she didn't have to map out a complicated eating plan or count calories or fat grams. The pounds came off and she has been able to keep them off ever since.

What works for Mary is a flexible strategy with very little structure. "I don't want to set myself up for failure by setting unattainable goals," she explains.

*****

Mary's Personal Plan

Section 1 - My Motivators

I want to live a long life and enjoy it
I want to feel good about myself
I want to enjoy shopping for new clothes
I try to focus on the positive results achieved rather than worrying about long-term maintenance

Section 2 - My Lame Excuses

I don't have time for a complicated diet
I don't want to prepare special meals for myself
I don't enjoy structure

Section 3 - I Can Resist Temptation

I won't keep sweets in the house to tempt me
I will stay busy so I don't focus on food
I can vicariously enjoy other people's enjoyment of food

Section 4 - My Ideal Weight

140 pounds

Section 5 - I Am A …

 koala

Section 6 - My Eating Strategies

Never eat anything sweet
Don't snack between meals
When eating out, share an entrée
Be conscious of when I've had enough food

Section 7 - My Exercise Program

I will go running with a friend three times/week
I will work out at a gym twice a week
I will play racquetball at every opportunity
I'll turn social interactions into opportunities for exercise

Section 8 - My Personal Tips

Drink lots of water
"Work out with a friend. Consider running or playing racquetball a social commitment rather than an exercise. Once I've agreed to meet a friend for some type of activity, I wouldn't dream of backing out. The time passes quickly and I enjoy it. Also, I recommend developing a variety of physical activities so you don't get burned out on a boring routine."

*****

Dennis C. recently lost 30 pounds through a modified Weight Watchers diet. When asked what his motivation was, he replied, "One day while I was in the grocery store parking lot waiting for my wife, I noticed a very obese woman struggling to get out of a large, presumably gas-guzzling vehicle. It occurred to me she wouldn't be able to squeeze into a normal-size car. To me, she represented the American "obesity epidemic" and I decided then and there I didn't want to be a part of it."

Dennis realized he needed to change his eating habits and lifestyle in order to maintain his weight loss. One of his techniques is to eat the same small breakfast and lunch each day, and then reward himself with more variety at dinnertime. A typical breakfast is one cup of cereal with skim milk. Lunch consists of a salad or lean meat with vegetables. Dinner might be a meal out, or fish and vegetables at home. He has discovered he likes eating healthy and the foods he is now eating are just as enjoyable as his old standbys of pasta, ribs, and fried foods.

Dennis's Personal Plan

Section 1 - My Motivators

I want to be healthy
I want people to see me as being in control
"I want to be around to enjoy my grandchildren someday. My old lifestyle increased my risk of various health problems and may have eventually affected my quality of life."

Section 2 - My Lame Excuses

I really enjoy food!

Section 3 - I Can Resist Temptation

I will allow myself some of my favorite foods
I will remind myself of my motivators
I will remember what I *don't* want to be like

Section 4 - My Ideal Weight

195 pounds

Section 5 - I Am A ...

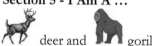 deer and gorilla

Section 6 - My Eating Strategies

Make trade-offs
Save my calories for later in the day
Splurge occasionally so I don't feel deprived
Fill up on protein

Section 7 - My Exercise Program

Do active things around the house instead of watching TV
Walk several times a week

Section 8 - My Personal Tips

Be very disciplined about eating a healthy breakfast and lunch
Limit between-meal snacking
"I don't want to give up the wine I enjoy with dinner, so I make trade-offs in other ways. Also, if I overdo it at a social event, I'll watch what I eat the next day to maintain an overall balance."

*****

When Raymond V. simultaneously reached the milestone numbers of 40 years old and 300 pounds, he decided he needed to reverse the trend. While he couldn't do anything about growing older, he was able to change his habits to take the weight off and improve his health. What worked for him was the Nutrisystem diet, which plans your meals and portion sizes for you. After losing 30 pounds and keeping it off, his formerly high cholesterol is now in the normal range.

Although the convenience of preplanned and prepackaged meals made losing weight easy, he had to develop better eating habits to keep it off. He now watches his portion sizes, never has second helpings, and tries to fill up on fruits and vegetables.

*****

Raymond's Personal Plan

Section 1 - My Motivators

I want to lower my cholesterol
I want to be healthy in general

I want to have improved physical endurance

Section 2 - My Lame Excuses

I like to be social at happy hours and other get-togethers
I don't want to have to think about what I eat
I like to relax

Section 3 - I Can Resist Temptation

I remind myself of my success in losing weight and I don't want to backslide
I will find other ways to enjoy a social life besides eating

Section 4 - My Ideal Weight

230 pounds

Section 5 - I Am A ...

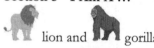 lion and gorilla

Section 6 - My Eating Strategies

Don't have second helpings
Control portion sizes
Try to eat healthy foods most of the time, but allow some exceptions

Section 7 - My Exercise Program

I will play golf as frequently as I can
I will participate in Scottish Games competitions
I will play sand volleyball
I will go to the gym regularly

Section 8 - My Personal Tips

"If you give in to temptation, don't just give up your whole eating plan. Get back into the program the next day and pick up where you left off."

*****

Vicki M. has never been heavy, but has struggled to keep from putting on pounds. Many of her family members have weight problems and she's afraid if she's not constantly vigilant, it will catch up with her too. She enjoys eating, drinking, and partying, but is determined to maintain an attractive and healthy weight.

Vicki has the discipline to plan her eating and exercise program. She buys low-calorie foods whenever possible and isn't afraid to try new products. She is a regular exerciser and also tries to build activity into her normal lifestyle. She drinks eight or more glasses of water per day to help keep her full and tries to watch her portion sizes.

*****

Vicki's Personal Plan

Section 1 - My Motivators

I want to avoid the high blood pressure and high cholesterol that run in my family
I want to wear trendy clothes and have them look good on me
I want to be strong
I want to maintain my weight so that I never have to go on an official diet

Section 2 - My Lame Excuses

I need to have a social life
I really enjoy high-calorie foods such as cheese, pasta, and wine

I'm not overweight so I can afford to binge occasionally

Section 3 - I Can Resist Temptation

I will substitute low-calorie products wherever possible
I won't keep junk food in the house
I will look at my own pictures of times when I looked my best

Section 4 - My Ideal Weight

132 pounds

Section 5 - I Am A ...

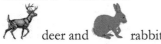 deer and   rabbit

Section 6 - My Eating Strategies

Make tradeoffs so I can have what I want sometimes
Use cooking spray instead of oil
Try to eat more protein and less carbs so I can stay full longer
and am less likely to snack
Save up calories for a special party or event

Section 7 - My Exercise Program

I will do a circuit workout three times/week
Walk to the gym, no matter what the weather is like
I will do calisthenics on Monday, Wednesday, Friday, and
Saturday each week
I will do a free weights routine three times a week
Ride a bicycle instead of driving a car

Section 8 - My Personal Tips

Get plenty of sleep—take an occasional "power nap"
Weigh myself every day and make a graph
Treat myself to a shopping spree if I have lost or maintained

my weight

Only eat one meal out per week

"One thing I do is to just stop buying junk. If it's there I'll eat it but if it's not, there's no way I'm going to run all the way to the store to get it, so eventually my craving passes."

*****

Elaine V. was raised with the "Polish" way of eating: her mother would fix a large amount of food, set it all out on the table, and dinner wasn't over until all the food was gone. It didn't matter how much food was prepared or how many people happened to be there—they all ate until there was nothing left. Although she managed to stay slim as a child and into her twenties, Elaine had gained weight in her thirties as a side effect of taking some medications for a health condition. In order to lose the weight, she had to "unlearn" the eating habits she had been taught as a child.

Elaine's strategy was two-fold: first, she stopped putting bowls of food on the table during meals. Instead she put small portions on her plate and left the rest of the food on the stove. One plate was all she allowed herself for each meal. Her second change was to have only two meals each day, usually breakfast and lunch, with no snacking between meals. The pounds started dropping rapidly and she has been able to keep them off. Now she will sometimes have three meals a day, but still controls portion sizes and avoids snacks.

*****

Elaine's Personal Plan

Section 1 - My Motivators

I want to be healthier

I want to be able to buy attractive clothes that fit me

Section 2 - My Lame Excuses

I hate to waste food
It's not my fault I gained weight; it's the medicine I'm taking

Section 3 - I Can Resist Temptation

I will look at pictures of myself when I was younger and slimmer
I will keep food out of my sight whenever possible

Section 4 - My Ideal Weight

145 pounds

Section 5 - I Am A ...

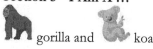gorilla and koala

Section 6 - My Eating Strategies

Eat a healthy breakfast and lunch and then skip supper
Use reasonable portion sizes
Eliminate snacking

Section 7 - My Exercise Program

I will go for walks whenever I can
I will lift hand weights and gradually increase the amount of the weights

Section 8 - My Personal Tips

Mix half diet and half regular soda instead of drinking all regular soda
Weigh myself only once a week
Never have second helpings

*****

You have seen how others have crafted unique plans to keep them healthy and slim for life. It's now up to you! Use the personal plan worksheet provided in Appendix A and fill in each section with your own strategies. Use any of the ideas presented here, borrow from the personal plans above, and feel free to invent your own strategies. Your plan can be as simple or as detailed as you like. You are the only one who needs to see it. And remember—by creating a plan that works for *you*, you too can live the thin life!

Part Six

Appendices

Appendix A

Personal Plan Worksheet

Here is the personal plan outline you can use to build your own plan. I've described each section throughout the book so that you could build your plan as you went along. However, don't worry if you didn't do that, it's not too late! Just get started right now.

You may choose to only use some parts of the plan or all of it. You can keep your plan very simple or you might decide to jot down every idea you want to try. It's all up to you. You decide what works best for you.

My Personal Plan

Section 1 - My Motivators

Section 2 - My Lame Excuses

Section 3 - I Can Resist Temptation

Section 4 - My Ideal Weight

Section 5 - I Am A ... (circle one or more)

 gorilla koala 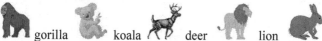 deer lion
rabbit

Section 6 - My Eating Strategies

Section 7 - My Exercise Program

Section 8 - My Personal Tips

Appendix B

Sample Food Logs

There are several ways of logging what you eat. Here are four examples you can choose from to see which works best for you. Each daily food log provides space for you to enter every item you eat, plus various counts depending on if you are watching your calories, fat, or carbs. Enter the date at the top of the page, and then start logging in everything you consume that day. I've allowed space for six meals, which gives you breakfast, lunch, and dinner, plus snacks for mid-morning, mid-afternoon, and after dinner. Don't feel you have to eat all six meals each day! You can always create your own form if your personal habits include fewer daily meals, or else just don't use all the lines.

The first example shown in Table B.1 is the most basic: the calorie log. Write down each food you eat, look up the number of calories for the amount you've eaten, then write in that number. At the end of the day, total up your calories and make sure they're within the limit you've set for yourself. Remember the calorie guidelines for maintaining your weight from Chapter 4:

- If you are sedentary or inactive: Multiply your current weight in pounds by 13
- If you are moderately active: Multiply your weight in pounds by 15

Elle Marie

- If you are very active: Multiply your weight in pounds by 17 to 19

It's a good idea to note your calorie limit on your log, then keep a running total throughout the day to make sure you don't exceed it. After you've done this for a while, you'll learn the number of calories in your typical foods so it will get easier and less time-consuming to track.

The next log, Table B.2, can be used if you are watching your fat intake. This is especially suited to the rabbit's eating style. For a low-fat diet, you should consume no more than 30% of your daily calories in the form of fat. This means you must track the number of fat grams consumed in addition to the number of calories. At the end of the day, use the formula provided at the bottom of the table to calculate the percentage of fat you have consumed for the day.

Next is the low carbohydrate food log, shown in Table B.3. This one is useful for lions. You will need to track your carb intake, and as a general rule try to keep it below 60 grams. You really should also watch your total calories, as there are many low-carb foods that have lots of calories and can still pack on the weight if you're not careful. I've included a column for tracking calories as well.

Table B.4 is my personal favorite. This is the type of daily food log I used when I dieted many years ago and successfully lost weight. It's a little more complicated than the others, but it's very effective. It's similar to the low-carb plan, but instead of tracking carbs, you track your protein intake and make sure it's at least 40% of your total calories. This high-protein diet is automatically low in carbohydrates. Enter in the foods eaten, then also track your protein grams and total calories. Use the formula at the bottom of the table to calculate your percentage of calories from protein.

The following pages have sample forms you can copy or use to create your own personal form.

Table B.1 - Calorie Counting Food Log Example

	Day:	Calories
Meal 1		
Meal 2		
Meal 3		
Meal 4		
Meal 5		
Meal 6		
	Total for the day	

Table B.2 - Fat Counting Food Log Example

Day:		Calories
Meal 1		
Meal 2		
Meal 3		
Meal 4		
Meal 5		
Meal 6		
	Total for the day	

% of calories from fat = (total fat grams x 9) / total calories
% of calories from fat should be no more than 30%

Table B.3 - Carb Counting Food Log Example

Day:		Carbs	Calories
Meal 1			
Meal 2			
Meal 3			
Meal 4			
Meal 5			
Meal 6			
	Totals for the day		

Total carbs should be less than 60 grams

Elle Marie

Table B.4 - High Protein Food Log Example

Day:		Protein	Calories
Meal 1			
Meal 2			
Meal 3			
Meal 4			
Meal 5			
Meal 6			
	Totals for the day		

% of calories from protein = (total protein grams x 4) / total calories

Appendix C

Recipes

I've done quite a bit of experimenting with recipes over the years. I like to take recipes from magazines, newspapers, books, and websites and then make adjustments to reduce the number of calories or fat and maybe add different seasonings for a change. While I'm interested in preparing healthy foods, I also want them to be tasty. All the recipes in this section are Elvis-tested and approved. Whenever I tell him I'm trying out a new dish, he grumbles about it and asks why I'm not making something that I already know he likes. But once he tries the new dish, nine times out of ten he loves it. I'm only including recipes for those dishes we both like. Well, okay, except for the recipes with cauliflower or asparagus.

Some of my tips for adapting recipes are to substitute applesauce for oil (especially when baking), substitute quick oats for breadcrumbs in meatballs or meatloaf, and substitute Splenda for sugar. You can use lower calorie margarine instead of butter, although that doesn't always work well for baked goods. My favorite is Smart Balance Olive Oil spread, which has only 60 calories per tablespoon, compared to 100 calories for butter or 120 calories for olive oil. It tastes great, cooks well, and also has healthy omega-3 oils in it.

When making pasta dishes, I like to reduce the amount of pasta by about half, but keep the other amounts the same.

This provides a saucier, more flavorful dish with fewer carbs.

For each recipe, I've listed the calorie, fat, carbohydrate, and protein counts to make it easier if you decide to try out my food logs.

So go ahead and try my recipes! And don't be afraid to change them to suit your own tastes. You'll notice there are lots of fish dishes listed, since fish is so versatile and low-calorie. Feel free to substitute chicken or another meat if you prefer. As long as you use lean meats, they'll still be healthy dishes. Enjoy!

Main Dishes

Teriyaki Salmon

1 1/2 lbs	salmon fillet
1 tbsp	olive oil
2 tbsp	teriyaki marinade
1/2 tsp	minced garlic
1/4 tsp	powdered ginger
2 tbsp	soy sauce
1 pkt	Splenda

1. Wash salmon and place in plastic bag.
2. In small bowl, mix oil, marinade, garlic, ginger, and soy sauce. Add to bag and marinate in refrigerator for 1 to 4 hours.
3. Broil salmon, skin side down, for 15 minutes.

Makes 4 servings. 280 calories, 14g fat, 2g carbs, 36g protein each

This is also delicious grilled.

Crab Mushroom Omelet

1 tbsp	Smart Balance spread with olive oil
1/2 cup	mushrooms, chopped
1/4 cup	onions, chopped
2 1/2 oz	imitation or real crab meat, shredded
1/2 cup	Egg Beaters
1/8 cup	skim milk
1/4 tsp	salt
1/4 tsp	pepper
1/4 cup	2% shredded cheese

1. Melt Smart Balance in small nonstick frying pan. Add mushrooms and onions and cook for 3 to 4 minutes. Add crabmeat and cook for another minute.
2. In small bowl, combine Egg Beaters, milk, salt, and pepper. Add egg mixture to pan, spreading evenly over crab and vegetables. Cook until bottom starts to brown.
3. Sprinkle cheese on top, then cook for one more minute. Fold over into crescent shape on plate.

Makes 1 serving. 310 calories, 13g fat, 16g carbs, 36g protein

Chicken Quesadilla

3 oz can	chicken breast
2 tbsp	salsa or picante sauce
1/4 cup	onions, chopped
1/4 cup	2% shredded cheese
2	low-carb tortillas
	cooking spray

1. Mix chicken, onion, salsa, and cheese in a small bowl. Spread mixture on one tortilla. Cover with remaining tortilla.
2. Spray cooking spray in non-stick frying pan and heat on medium heat. Add quesadilla to pan. Cook until bottom tortilla is browned.
3. Spray cooking spray on top of quesadilla, then flip to other side. Cook until browned.

Makes 1 serving. 310 calories, 10g fat, 21g carbs, 30g protein

Easy Tuna Melt

3 oz. can	light tuna
2	low-carb tortillas
1/4 cup	2% shredded cheese
	cooking spray

1. Drain tuna and spread on one tortilla. Sprinkle with cheese. Cover with remaining tortilla.
2. Spray cooking spray in non-stick frying pan and heat on medium heat. Add tuna tortilla to pan. Cook until bottom tortilla is browned.
3. Spray cooking spray on top of tortilla, then flip to other side. Cook until browned.

Makes 1 serving. 310 calories, 10g fat, 15g carbs, 35g protein

Chinese Grilled Fish

4	pieces flaky white fish, such as tilapia or orange roughy (6 ounces each)
1 tsp	peanut oil
1 tsp	minced garlic
1/2 tsp	crushed red pepper flakes
1/2 tsp	Chinese 5-spice powder
1/4 tsp	ground ginger
2 tbsp	soy sauce
1 pkt	Splenda

1. Wash and debone fish if necessary. Place fish in zip-top bag.
2. Mix oil, garlic, pepper flakes, Chinese 5-spice powder, ginger, soy sauce, and Splenda in a small bowl. Pour into bag over fish. Marinate in refrigerator for 1 to 3 hours.
3. Place fish on heated grill. Pour remaining marinade over fish. Grill on low heat for 5 to 6 minutes on each side.

Makes 4 servings. 135 calories, 2g fat, .5g carbs, 25g protein each

This is one of Elvis's all time favorites.

Tarragon Breaded Cod

1 tbsp	cornmeal
1 tbsp	flour
1 tbsp	tarragon
1 tsp	salt
4	cod fish fillets (6 ounces each)
2 tbsp	Smart Balance spread

1.   Combine cornmeal, flour, tarragon, and salt. Coat fish fillets with cornmeal mixture.
2.   Melt Smart Balance in a non-stick skillet over medium high heat. Add fish and cook 4 to 6 minutes on each side.

Makes 4 servings. 165 calories, 5g fat, 3g carbs, 25g protein each

Another Elvis favorite! You can substitute other spices, such as chili powder, for the tarragon.

Easy Italian Grilled Fish

4	fish fillets (6 ounces each)
1/3 cup	low-calorie Italian dressing
1 tbsp	lemon juice
1/4 tsp	pepper
1/4 tsp	paprika

1.　Mix dressing, lemon juice, pepper, and paprika in a bowl or zip-top bag. Add fish and marinate 1 to 3 hours.

2.　Grill on barbecue or broil in oven for 5 to 7 minutes per side.

Makes 4 servings. 140 calories, 3g fat, 1g carbs, 25g protein each

Shrimp Scampi

2 tbsp	olive oil
1 tbsp	minced garlic
1/4 tsp	paprika
1 tbsp	parsley
1/2 tsp	salt
1/2 tsp	pepper
1 1/2 lbs	large shrimp, peeled and deveined

1. Combine oil, garlic, paprika, salt, pepper, and parsley in a bowl. Add shrimp and toss well. Cover and refrigerate for 1 hour.
2. Turn broiler on high heat.
3. Thread shrimp onto skewers. Brush with marinade.
4. Broil shrimp for 3 to 4 minutes, turning once. You can also put the skewers on a hot grill for 4 to 5 minutes on each side.

Makes 4 servings. 135 calories, 8g fat, 2g carbs, 13g protein each

Curry Battered Fish

4	fish fillets (6 ounces each)
1/2 tsp	salt
1/2 tsp	pepper
1 tsp	ground turmeric
1 1/2 tsp	curry powder
1/4 tsp	cayenne pepper
2 tbsp	peanut or vegetable oil
3/4 cup	flour
3/4 cup	warm water

1. Combine all spices in a small bowl, then rub into both sides of fish.
2. Heat 1 tablespoon of oil on medium high in a large non-stick skillet.
3. Combine flour with warm water to make a batter about the consistency of yogurt.
4. Turn heat up to high. Dip each piece of fish into batter, letting excess batter drip off, then place in pan. Cook 5 to 8 minutes on each side, until coating is golden and crispy.

Makes 4 servings. 260 calories, 8g fat, 18g carbs, 27g protein each

It's hard to believe this crispy fried fish is so low in calories.

Mexican Meatloaf for Two

1/2 lb	ground beef
1 jar	mild salsa or picante sauce (8 ounces)
1/2 cup	Egg Beaters
1/4 cup	rolled oats
1 tsp	cumin
1/2 tsp	salt
1/4 tsp	pepper
1/2 cup	green peppers, diced

1. Preheat oven to 450°.
2. Mix salsa, Egg Beaters, oats, cumin, salt and pepper in large bowl. Stir in peppers. Add ground beef and mix well.
3. Form mixture into 2 loaves, about 6 inches by 3 inches each. Place on baking sheet.
4. Bake for 20 minutes.

Makes 2 generous servings. 410 calories, 24g fat, 18g carbs, 27g protein each

Elvis likes to put a dollop of sour cream on his meatloaf.

Chili-Rubbed Salmon

1 tbsp	olive oil
4	salmon fillets (6 ounces each)
3/4 tsp	chili powder
1/8 tsp	cayenne pepper
3 tsp	brown sugar
3/4 tsp	cumin
1/2 tsp	salt

1. Preheat broiler.
2. Brush oil on salmon.
3. In a small bowl, mix together chili powder, pepper, brown sugar, cumin and salt. Rub into salmon.
4. Broil for 10 to 12 minutes.

Makes 4 servings. 280 calories, 14g fat, 4g carbs, 36g protein each

Sweet and spicy is a great combination!

Spiced Baked Chicken

4	boneless, skinless chicken breasts (about 6 ounces each)
1 tsp	crushed rosemary
1/2 tsp	thyme
1/2 tsp	onion powder
1/2 tsp	salt
1/2 tsp	pepper
1/4 tsp	garlic powder
1/8 tsp	cinnamon
1 tbsp	olive oil

1. Preheat oven to 400°.
2. Mix all spices in a small bowl.
3. Brush chicken breasts lightly with olive oil. Sprinkle with spices on all sides. Place chicken in baking dish.
4. Bake for 20 to 25 minutes.

Makes 4 servings. 305 calories, 9g fat, 0g carbs, 52g protein each

Chicken Crescent Casserole

3 cups	chicken breast, cooked
1 can	reduced fat cream of chicken soup (10 ¾ oz)
1/2 cup	light mayonnaise
1/2 cup	light sour cream
1 can	reduced fat crescent roll dough (8 rolls)
1 tbsp	Smart Balance, melted
2 tbsp	Parmesan cheese, shredded or grated
	cooking spray

1. Preheat oven to 375°. Spray a 9x13-inch baking dish with nonstick cooking spray.
2. Shred or dice chicken into small pieces. Mix chicken, soup, mayonnaise, and sour cream in a large bowl. Transfer to baking dish.
3. Bake for 25 minutes, then remove from oven.
4. Unroll dough and spread on top of chicken mixture. Brush melted Smart Balance over dough.
5. Return to oven and bake for an additional 10 to 12 minutes.
6. Remove from oven. Sprinkle with Parmesan cheese and bake for 1 to 2 more minutes.

Makes 8 servings. 180 calories, 12g fat, 4g carbs, 18g protein each

Elvis always ask for seconds of this casserole! At only 180 calories per serving, why not?

Salmon in Curry Sauce

3/4 lb	salmon fillet
1/4 tsp	salt
1/8 tsp	pepper
1 tbsp	Dijon mustard
1/4 cup	plain nonfat yogurt
2 tsp	curry powder
	olive oil cooking spray

1. Preheat oven to 400°.
2. Spray baking tray with olive oil. Place salmon in tray, skin side down.
3. Spray salmon with olive oil and sprinkle with salt and pepper.
4. Roast on middle shelf of oven for about 12 to 15 minutes.
5. While salmon is cooking, combine mustard, yogurt, and curry powder in a small bowl to make a sauce.
6. Remove salmon from oven and immediately spread it with sauce.

Makes 2 servings. 285 calories, 13g fat, 4g carbs, 36g protein each

Curry powder has antioxidant properties, making this a very healthy dish.

Briny Herb Chicken

4	boneless, skinless chicken breasts (about 6 ounces each)
1/4 cup	salt
1/4 cup	brown sugar
2	whole bay leaves
1 cup	hot water
3 cups	cold water
1	lemon, sliced
1	small onion, sliced
1 tsp	minced garlic

1. Place salt, sugar, and bay leaves in a large bowl. Add hot water and mix until salt and sugar are fully dissolved. Stir in cold water and let the brine come to room temperature.
2. Add lemon, onion, garlic, and chicken breasts. Cover with plastic wrap and refrigerate for 2 hours.
3. Preheat grill. Remove chicken from brine. Grill over high heat for 6 to 8 minutes on each side.

Makes 4 servings. 190 calories, 4g fat, 2g carbs, 34g protein each

The brine tenderizes the chicken as well as adding flavor.

Spicy Latin Pork Roast

2 lbs	boneless pork loin roast
1 tbsp	chili powder
1/2 tsp	cayenne pepper
3/4 tsp	cinnamon
1 tsp	salt
2 tsp	ground cumin
1 1/2 tsp	ground coriander
1 tsp	black pepper
2 tsp	brown sugar

1. Preheat oven to 350°.
2. Blend sugar and all spices in a small bowl. Rub evenly over pork.
3. Bake for 40 to 50 minutes. Let stand 10 minutes before slicing.

Makes 8 servings. 215 calories, 12g fat, 1g carbs, 23g protein each

One-Dish Beef Stroganoff

1 lb	boneless beef sirloin steak
1/2 tsp	minced garlic
1	small onion, chopped
1 can	beef broth (14 oz)
8 oz	mushrooms, sliced
1/2 tsp	salt
1/2 tsp	paprika
2 cups	uncooked medium egg noodles
1/2 cup	light sour cream
1 tsp	dried parsley (or 1 tbsp fresh chopped parsley)

1.   Slice beef into thin strips. In nonstick skillet over medium high heat, cook beef, garlic, and onion for 5 minutes.
2.   Stir in broth, mushrooms, salt and paprika. Bring to a boil. Add noodles. Cover and cook over low heat for 10 minutes, stirring often.
3.   Stir in sour cream and heat through but do not let it come to a boil. Sprinkle with parsley and serve.

Makes 4 servings. 290 calories, 9g fat, 21g carbs, 28g protein each

Garlic Rosemary Fish

4	fish fillets (6 ounces each)
2 tsp	minced garlic
2 tsp	dried rosemary
2 tbsp	olive oil
2 tsp	salt
1 tsp	pepper
1/4 cup	Smart Balance spread, melted
2 tbsp	lemon juice

1. Stir together garlic, rosemary, oil, salt, and pepper. Rub evenly over fish. Cover and refrigerate for 1 hour.
2. Grill fish over medium heat 5 to 7 minutes on each side.
3. Mix melted Smart Balance and lemon juice and pour over fish.

Makes 4 servings. 250 calories, 15g fat, 2g carbs, 25g protein each

Chili Crusted Fish

3/4 lb	white fish fillets, such as orange roughy or tilapia
2 tbsp	flour
1 tsp	ground cumin
1 tsp	chili powder
1/2 tsp	salt
1/4 tsp	pepper
1/4 cup	Egg Beaters
1 tbsp	olive oil

1.   Mix flour and spices in a shallow bowl.
2.   Pour Egg Beaters in a separate shallow bowl.
3.   Dip fish in Egg Beaters, then in flour mixture, coating both sides. Shake off excess flour.
4.   Heat oil in a nonstick skillet over medium high heat. Sauté fish 4 to 5 minutes on each side.

Makes 2 servings. 220 calories, 8g fat, 7g carbs, 29g protein each

Low-fat Meatloaf

1 lb	lean ground beef
1/2 can	low-fat cream of mushroom soup
1/4 cup	rolled oats
1/2 cup	Egg Beaters
1	small onion, chopped
1/2 pkg	onion soup mix

1. Preheat oven to 375°.
2. Mix together mushroom soup, Egg Beaters, and oats in large bowl.
3. Stir in onion soup mix and chopped onions.
4. Add ground beef and mix well.
5. Form into loaf on baking sheet. Bake for 1 hour.

Makes 4 servings. 325 calories, 17g fat, 14g carbs, 26g protein each

Salmon Parmesan

1 1/4 lbs	salmon fillet
1/4 cup	light mayonnaise
2 tbsp	Parmesan cheese, grated
2 tbsp	fresh chives, chopped
1 tsp	Worcestershire sauce
	cooking spray

1. Preheat oven to 450°.
2. Spray baking sheet with nonstick cooking spray. Place fish on sheet.
3. Stir together mayonnaise, cheese, 1 tablespoon chives, and Worcestershire sauce in small bowl.
4. Spread mayonnaise mixture over fish.
5. Bake uncovered for about 15 minutes. Sprinkle on remaining chives and serve.

Makes 4 servings. 260 calories, 16g fat, 0g carbs, 32g protein each

Spicy Shrimp

1 1/2 lbs	shrimp, peeled and deveined
1/2 tsp	salt
1/4 tsp	pepper
1/4 cup	Smart Balance spread
1	medium onion, chopped
1/2 tsp	minced garlic
1/8 tsp	crushed red pepper flakes
1 can	tomato sauce (14 oz)
1/2 cup	chicken broth

1. Season shrimp with salt and pepper.
2. Melt Smart Balance in nonstick skillet over medium high heat.
3. Add shrimp and cook for 3 to 4 minutes, turning once. Remove shrimp and keep warm.
4. In same skillet, cook onion for about 4 minutes. Stir in garlic and pepper flakes and cook for an additional 30 seconds.
5. Add tomato sauce and chicken broth. Bring to a boil over high heat.
6. Reduce heat to low and simmer for 3 minutes.
7. Return shrimp to skillet and heat through.

Makes 4 servings. 167 calories, 8g fat, 10g carbs, 13g protein each

Lemon Ginger Chicken

4	boneless, skinless chicken breasts (about 6 ounces each)
2 tsp	cornstarch
1 tbsp	soy sauce
1/4 cup	soy sauce
1/4 cup	lemon juice
1/4 cup	fat-free chicken broth
1 tsp	ground ginger
1 tsp	minced garlic
1 tbsp	Splenda
1 tbsp	olive oil

1. Mix 1 teaspoon cornstarch and 1 tablespoon soy sauce in a medium mixing bowl. Add chicken breasts and marinate in refrigerator for 10 minutes.
2. Stir lemon juice, 1/4 cup soy sauce, chicken broth, ginger, garlic, Splenda and remaining 1 teaspoon cornstarch together in a separate mixing bowl.
3. Heat oil in a medium-sized frying pan.
4. Add chicken to pan and cook over medium high heat for 4 to 5 minutes on each side.
5. Add sauce and cook for an additional 1 to 2 minutes.

Makes 4 servings. 305 calories, 9g fat, 3g carbs, 49g protein each

Spicy Mustard Fish

4	fish fillets (6 ounces each)
1 tsp	cumin
1/2 tsp	salt
1/4 tsp	pepper
2 tbsp	spicy brown mustard
1 tbsp	Smart Balance, melted
	cooking spray

1. Preheat oven to 400°.
2. Spray baking sheet with cooking spray. Place fish on baking sheet.
3. Brush fish with melted Smart Balance. Dust with cumin, salt, and pepper. Spread mustard over the fish.
4. Place baking sheet in oven and bake fish for 4 to 6 minutes on each side.

Makes 4 servings. 250 calories, 6g fat, 2g carbs, 44g protein each

Quick, easy, and delicious!

Parmesan Garlic Chicken

4	boneless, skinless chicken breasts (about 6 ounces each)
1/4 cup	Parmesan cheese, grated
1 pkt	roasted garlic salad dressing mix (8-serving size)
	cooking spray

1. Preheat oven to 400°.
2. Mix cheese and salad dressing mix in a small bowl.
3. Moisten chicken with water, then coat with cheese mixture.
4. Spray shallow baking dish with cooking spray. Place chicken in dish. Put dish in oven and bake for 20 to 25 minutes.

Makes 4 servings. 285 calories, 8g fat, 2g carbs, 49g protein each

Tequila Lime Chicken

4	boneless, skinless chicken breasts (about 6 ounces each)
1/3 cup	lime juice
1/3 cup	water
3 tbsp	tequila
1 tbsp	Splenda
1 tbsp	soy sauce
1 tsp	minced garlic
1 tbsp	olive oil

1.   Combine lime juice, water, tequila, Splenda, soy sauce, and garlic in a zip-top plastic bag. Add chicken and refrigerate for at least 2 hours.
2.   Drain chicken, discarding marinade. Brush with olive oil.
3.   Preheat grill on high heat. Grill chicken over hot fire for about 10 minutes on each side.

Makes 4 servings. 310 calories, 9g fat, 3g carbs, 47g protein each

Cranberry Pork Roast

2 1/2 lbs	rolled pork loin roast
1 can	jellied cranberry sauce (16 oz)
1/2 cup	Splenda
1/2 cup	cranberry juice
1 tsp	dry mustard
1/4 tsp	ground cloves
1 tsp	salt
2 tbsp	cornstarch
2 tbsp	cold water

1. Place pork roast in a slow cooker.
2. In a medium bowl, mash cranberry sauce. Stir in Splenda, cranberry juice, mustard, cloves, and salt. Pour mixture over roast.
3. Cover and cook on low for 6 to 8 hours.
4. Remove roast and keep warm.
5. Skim fat from juices. Measure 2 cups of the remaining liquid into saucepan, adding extra water if necessary to make 2 cups. Bring to a boil over medium high heat.
6. Combine the cornstarch and cold water in a small bowl to make a smooth paste; stir into gravy in pan. Cook, stirring, until thickened. Serve over sliced pork.

Makes 8 servings. 360 calories, 15g fat, 23g carbs, 28g protein each

Mini Frittatas

1/4 lb	Swiss cheese, finely chopped
1/4 lb	ham, finely chopped
4 cups	Egg Beaters
1 tbsp	half-and-half
3 tsp	dried chives, chopped (or 3 tbsp fresh)
1/2 tsp	salt
1/4 tsp	pepper
dash	hot sauce
	cooking spray

1. Preheat oven to 375°.
2. Spray 12-muffin tin with cooking spray. Scatter cheese and ham evenly among the cups.
3. Mix Egg Beaters, half-and-half, chives, salt, and pepper in mixing bowl. Add hot sauce to taste.
4. Fill muffin cups to just below the rim with egg mixture. Bake for 12 to 15 minutes.

Makes 6 servings (2 frittatas each). 210 calories, 7g fat, 4g carbs, 26g protein per serving

Vegetables and Side Dishes

Creamed Spinach

12 oz bag	fresh spinach leaves
1 tbsp	Smart Balance spread
2 tbsp	powdered garlic herb soup mix
3 oz	light cream cheese, softened
2 tbsp	light sour cream

1. Melt Smart Balance in skillet on medium heat.
2. Add spinach and cook until just wilted.
3. Sprinkle on salad dressing mix and stir in.
4. Add cream cheese and sour cream and heat until melted, blending well.

Makes 4 servings. 105 calories, 7g fat, 7g carbs, 5g protein each

Even people who don't usually like vegetables love this dish.

Carrot Coins

1	bunch fresh carrots (about ½ pound)
1 tbsp	Smart Balance spread
1/2 tsp	salt
1 tsp	parsley
1 pkt	Splenda

1. Peel carrots and cut off ends. Chop into round pieces about 1/4 inch thick.
2. Steam carrots in vegetable steamer according to steamer instructions, or microwave with 2 tablespoons water for 5 minutes.
3. Add Smart Balance, parsley, salt, and Splenda to cooked carrots. Mix well and serve.

Makes 2 servings. 125 calories, 4g fat, 21g carbs, 2g protein

This easy recipe is a family favorite.

Mashed Cauliflower

4 cups	fresh cauliflower florets
1/2 cup	light sour cream
1/2 tsp	salt
1 tbsp	Smart Balance spread

1. Cut cauliflower florets into small pieces and place in microwave-safe bowl. Add a few tablespoons of water.
2. Microwave for 5 minutes on high. Drain water.
3. Mash cauliflower as finely as possible. Mix in sour cream, salt, and Smart Balance until creamy.

Makes 4 servings. 85 calories, 5g fat, 8g carbs, 3g protein each

I must admit Elvis won't eat cauliflower and he wanted me to take this recipe out. However, I love it and it's so low calorie and healthy!

Spinach Feta Orzo

3/4 cup	orzo
1 1/2 tbsp	olive oil
1 1/2 tsp	minced garlic
1/4 tsp	crushed red pepper
3	green onions, chopped
10 oz	fresh spinach leaves (or thawed, chopped frozen spinach)
1 tbsp	lemon juice
1/2 tsp	salt
1/2 cup	crumbled feta cheese

1. Boil water in a saucepan. Add orzo and boil uncovered for about 8 or 9 minutes.
2. While the orzo is cooking, heat oil in a large skillet over high heat.
3. Reduce heat to medium. Add garlic, red pepper, and onions. Cook for 2 minutes.
4. Add spinach and cook for an additional 4 minutes.
5. Drain pasta and add to spinach mixture. Toss in lemon juice, salt, and feta cheese. Stir well.

Makes 4 servings. 230 calories, 10g fat, 27g carbs, 8g protein each

Mashed Sweet Potatoes

2	large sweet potatoes
1/2 cup	unsweetened applesauce
1/2 tsp	cinnamon
1/2 tsp	salt

1. Wash sweet potatoes and pierce in several places with fork.
2. Microwave potatoes on paper towels on high for 15 minutes, turning halfway through.
3. Remove skins. Mash potatoes in large bowl, then stir in applesauce, cinnamon, and salt.
4. Microwave on high for 5 additional minutes. Stir and serve.

Makes 4 servings. 95 calories, 0g fat, 22g carbs, 1g protein each

Fettuccini with Mushrooms

4 oz	fettuccini
2 tsp	Smart Balance
1 1/2 cups	mushrooms, sliced
1	small onion, chopped
1/2 tsp	garlic
1 tbsp	skim milk
1/3 cup	Parmesan cheese, grated

1. Heat water to boiling in saucepan. Add fettuccini and cook according to package directions.
2. While fettuccini is cooking, heat Smart Balance in a separate pan. Add mushrooms, onion, and garlic. Cook until onions are tender.
3. Drain fettuccini, then add to mushrooms and onions. Add milk and Parmesan cheese. Toss gently until fettuccini is well coated.

Makes 4 servings. 175 calories, 5g fat, 24g carbs, 9g protein each

Pasta Primavera

1 tbsp	Smart Balance
1 1/2 tsp	minced garlic
1	small onion, chopped
2 cups	broccoli florets
2 cups	uncooked bowtie pasta
1/4 cup	Romano or Parmesan cheese, grated
6 oz	ricotta cheese
1/2 tsp	salt
1/4 tsp	red pepper flakes
2 tbsp	cream

1. Melt Smart Balance in a medium pan over medium heat. Add garlic and onion and sauté for 3 to 4 minutes.
2. Bring water to a boil in a separate pan over medium high heat. Add broccoli. When water returns to a boil, add pasta and cook for 10 to 12 minutes.
3. Drain pasta and broccoli, then add to onions and garlic. Add cheeses, seasonings, and cream. Stir well. Simmer until cheese melts.

Makes 4 servings. 225 calories, 10g fat, 23g carbs, 13g protein each

Green Beans Italiano

2 1/2 cups	fresh green beans
1 tbsp	olive oil
1/2 cup	mushrooms, sliced
2 tbsp	onions, chopped
1/2 tsp	minced garlic
1/4 tsp	Italian seasoning
1/2 tsp	salt
1/4 tsp	pepper

1. Steam green beans in vegetable steamer according to steamer instructions, or microwave with 2 tablespoons water for 5 minutes.
2. In large skillet, heat oil over medium high heat. Add mushrooms, onions, and garlic and sauté for 4 to 5 minutes.
3. Drain green beans and add to skillet. Add Italian seasoning, salt, and pepper and mix well.

Makes 4 servings. 60 calories, 4g fat, 6g carbs, 2g protein each

Broccoli au Gratin

1 lb	broccoli florets (about 4 cups)
1/4 cup	Smart Balance spread
1/4 cup	flour
1 1/2 cups	skim milk
1 1/2 tsp	dry mustard
1 tsp	salt
1/4 tsp	black pepper
1/8 tsp	cayenne pepper
1/8 tsp	nutmeg
1/4 cup	breadcrumbs
1/4 cup	Parmesan cheese, grated
1 tbsp	olive oil

1. Preheat oven to 350°.
2. Bring a large pot of water to a boil. Add broccoli; cook until it begins to soften, about 3 minutes. Remove broccoli from pot and place in a large bowl.
3. Melt Smart Balance in a medium saucepan. Add flour and whisk until blended. Add milk. Whisk continuously until sauce comes to a boil. Add mustard, salt, peppers, and nutmeg. Cook at a low boil for several minutes, stirring constantly.
4. Pour sauce over broccoli and stir to mix completely. Pour into casserole dish.
5. In a bowl, combine breadcrumbs and grated cheese. Add olive oil and mix with fork.
6. Top casserole with crumb mixture.
7. Bake for 30 to 35 minutes.

Makes 6 servings. 175 calories, 9g fat, 17g carbs, 9g protein each

Garlic Herb Mixed Vegetables

1/2 lb	broccoli florets
1/2 lb	cauliflower florets
1 tbsp	Smart Balance spread
1/2 tsp	salt
1 tsp	Mrs. Dash Garlic & Herb seasoning blend

1. Steam broccoli and cauliflower in vegetable steamer according to steamer instructions, or microwave with 2 tablespoons water for 5 minutes.
2. Add Smart Balance, salt, and seasoning blend. Stir well and serve immediately.

Makes 4 servings. 35 calories, 2g fat, 4g carbs, 2g protein each

Cheesy Spicy Zucchini

4	small zucchini
4 oz	light cream cheese, softened
1/2 cup	pepper jack cheese, shredded
1/2 cup	Parmesan cheese, shredded
1/4 tsp	cayenne pepper
1 tsp	dried chives
	cooking spray

1. Preheat oven to 350°.
2. Slice zucchini in half lengthwise. Blanch in boiling salted water for 2 minutes.
3. Drain, then place zucchini in a bowl of ice to cool. Remove from ice and blot dry with paper towels.
4. Hollow out zucchini, leaving at least a 1/4 inch wall.
5. Combine cheeses, pepper, and chives in mixing bowl. Stuff zucchini with cheese mixture.
6. Spray baking dish with cooking spray, then place zucchini in dish.
7. Bake for 8 to 10 minutes.

Makes 4 servings. 210 calories, 16g fat, 5g carbs, 13g protein each

Almond Asparagus

2 tbsp	sliced almonds
1 lb	fresh asparagus
1/2 cup	water
1 tbsp	Smart Balance spread
1 tbsp	lemon juice
1/2 tsp	salt
1/4 tsp	pepper

1. Place almonds on a plate. Toast in microwave on high for 1 minute.
2. Cut asparagus into 1-inch pieces. In a skillet, simmer asparagus in water for 6 minutes (crisp) to 10 minutes (tender).
3. Drain water. Stir in Smart Balance, lemon juice, salt, and pepper.
4. Serve topped with toasted almonds.

Makes 4 servings. 50 calories, 3g fat, 5g carbs, 0g protein each

Creamy Mashed Potatoes

3-4	medium potatoes (about 2 lbs)
1 1/4 cups	chicken broth
2 tsp	minced garlic
1 tsp	salt
1/4 tsp	pepper
dash	hot pepper sauce
1/4 cup	light sour cream
4 tsp	dried parsley, chopped (or 4 tbsp fresh)

1. Cut potatoes into 1-inch cubes and place in saucepan. Add chicken broth, garlic, salt, pepper, and hot sauce.
2. Bring to a boil over medium high heat. Reduce heat and cover. Cook for 20 to 25 minutes stirring occasionally until broth is absorbed and potatoes are soft.
3. Remove potatoes from heat and mash. Stir in sour cream. Sprinkle with parsley and serve.

Makes 6 servings. 95 calories, 1g fat, 18g carbs, 3g protein each

Desserts

Low-fat Mini Cheesecakes

8 oz	light cream cheese, softened
8 oz	part-skim ricotta cheese
1/2 cup	Splenda
1/2 tsp	almond extract
3	egg whites
36	mini vanilla wafers

1. Preheat oven to 350°.
2. In a large mixing bowl, combine cream cheese and ricotta until well blended. Add Splenda and almond extract, mixing well.
3. In another mixing bowl, beat egg whites until soft peaks form. Fold egg whites gradually into cheese mixture until well combined.
4. Place one vanilla wafer in each cup of a mini muffin tin. Fill cups about 3/4 full with egg cheese mixture (about 1 level tablespoon).
5. Bake muffins for 17 to 18 minutes.

Makes 36 mini muffins. 35 calories, 2g fat, 2g carbs, 2g protein per muffin

Elle Marie

Marble Brownies

1 pkg	light/reduced calorie brownie mix (20-ounce box)
8 oz	fat free cream cheese, softened
1/3 cup	Splenda
1/4 cup	Egg Beaters
1/2 tsp	vanilla
1/2 cup	semi-sweet chocolate chips

1. Preheat oven to 350°.
2. Prepare brownie mix as directed on package. Pour into greased 9x13-inch baking pan.
3. Beat cream cheese and Splenda in small bowl with electric mixer on medium speed until well blended. Add Egg Beaters and vanilla; mix well.
4. Pour cream cheese mixture over brownie batter. Cut through batter with knife several times for marble effect. Sprinkle with chocolate chips.
5. Bake 35 to 40 minutes or until cream cheese is lightly browned. Cool and cut into 18 squares.

Makes 18 brownies. 175 calories, 4g fat, 33g carbs, 3g protein each

Moist Muffins

1 pkg	cake mix (any flavor)
1 can	pumpkin (15 ounces)
1/2 cup	water

1. Preheat oven to 350°.
2. Place pumpkin in mixing bowl. Mix in cake mix. Add water and stir until batter is pourable. Add a little more water if necessary.
3. Line muffin pans with paper muffin cups. Pour batter into muffin pans.
4. Bake for 20 to 25 minutes.

Makes 24 muffins. 128 calories, 2g fat, 18g carbs, 1g protein each

Chocolate Cheesecake

16 oz   light cream cheese, softened (2 8-ounce packages)
1/3 cup   Splenda
1 1/2 tsp   vanilla extract
2   eggs
1/2 cup   heavy cream
1 box   sugar-free chocolate instant pudding mix (4-serving size)

1. Preheat oven to 350°.
2. Mix softened cream cheese, Splenda, vanilla, and eggs in a mixing bowl.
3. In a separate bowl, whisk cream and pudding mix until smooth. Add to cream cheese mixture. Mix on high until blended.
4. Pour batter into pie pan and bake for 40 minutes.
5. Refrigerate for at least 3 hours.

Makes 8 servings. 195 calories, 14g fat, 8g carbs, 8g protein each

Incredible Strawberry Pie

2 cups	water
1 pkg	sugar free cook-n-serve vanilla pudding
1 pkg	sugar free strawberry Jell-O
4 cups	strawberries
8 oz	Cool Whip

1. Place water and pudding mix in a saucepan and bring to a boil over medium high heat. Remove from stove.
2. Add Jell-O and stir. Let cool.
3. Clean and slice the fresh strawberries.
4. Line a pie plate with strawberries. Pour cooled pudding on top. Allow to set in refrigerator for at least one hour or until firm.
5. Top with Cool Whip and serve.

Makes 6 servings. 135 calories, 4g fat, 24g carbs, 2g protein each

Elle Marie

Raisin Apple Dessert for One

1	medium apple, sliced thin
1 tsp	Smart Balance spread, melted
2 tbsp	cinnamon
2 pkts	Splenda
1 tbsp	raisins

1. Place apple slices in microwave safe dish. Pour melted Smart Balance over apple.
2. Combine cinnamon and Splenda. Stir in raisins.
3. Sprinkle raisin mixture over apple slices.
4. Cover and microwave on high for 2 to 3 minutes or until apple slices are tender.

Makes 1 serving. 130 calories, 2g fat, 28g carbs, 0g protein

Cinnamon Crisp Tortillas

2	low-fat 8-inch flour tortillas
2 tsp	Smart Balance spread, melted
1/2 tsp	cinnamon
1/2 tsp	sugar

1. Preheat broiler.
2. Arrange tortillas on nonstick baking sheet. Brush each tortilla with 1 tsp of the melted Smart Balance.
3. Combine cinnamon with sugar and sprinkle 1/2 tsp of the mixture on each tortilla.
4. Broil on lowest rack 1 to 2 minutes.

Makes 2 servings. 125 calories, 5g fat, 19g carbs, 2g protein each

Elle Marie

Pumpkin Fluff

1 cup	canned pumpkin
1 tsp	pumpkin pie spice
1 cup	skim milk
1 cup	Cool Whip topping
1 pkg	sugar-free fat-free vanilla instant pudding mix

1. Mix together pumpkin, spice, and milk until well blended.
2. Add pudding mix. Beat by hand for 2 minutes.
3. Fold in Cool Whip.
4. Refrigerate for at least 30 minutes.

Makes 4 servings. 130 calories, 5g fat, 18g carbs, 3g protein each

For Thanksgiving, use pumpkin fluff as a filling in a low-fat graham cracker pie crust.

Strawberry Cream Cheese Shortcake

5 cups	sliced strawberries
1/4 cup	Splenda
8 oz	fat free cream cheese, softened
1/2 cup	powdered sugar
8 oz	Cool Whip
1	angel food cake, broken into pieces

1. Mix Splenda into sliced strawberries and set aside.
2. Beat cream cheese and powdered sugar. Fold in Cool Whip and cake cubes.
3. Spread into a 9x13-inch pan. Cover and chill for 2 hours.
4. Before serving, spread sweetened, sliced strawberries on top and top each serving with a dollop of Cool Whip.

Makes 12 servings. 220 calories, 2g fat, 44g carbs, 6g protein each

Banana Split Cake

1	prepared angel food cake
1 pkg	fat-free, sugar-free Jell-O instant pudding
2 cups	skim milk
4	medium bananas
4 cups	strawberries
2 tubs	Cool Whip (8 ounces each)

1. Prepare the pudding with skim milk as directed on the box.
2. Cut bananas and strawberries into bite-sized pieces.
3. Cut or tear the angel food cake into bite-sized pieces.
4. Separate all ingredients in half. Layer ingredients in the following order: half of the angel food cake, half of the pudding, half of the bananas, half of the cool whip, half of the strawberries.
5. Repeat the layer with the second half of ingredients.

Makes 12 servings. 255 calories, 4g fat, 51g carbs, 5g protein each

Lemon Sponge Bars

1 pkg	angel food cake mix (one-step mix kind)
1 can	lemon pie filling (22 ounces)
1 tsp	Smart Balance spread

1. Preheat oven to 350°.
2. Mix lemon pie filling with dry angel food cake mix in large bowl.
3. Rub Smart Balance in a 15x10-inch jelly roll pan. Pour in cake batter and bake for 25 minutes.
4. Cool and cut into 20 bars.

Makes 20 bars. 135 calories, 1g fat, 29g carbs, 2g protein each

You can also use a large cookie sheet instead of a jelly roll pan.

Appendix D

Bibliography

Chapter 1

1. L. Carrel; H.F. Willard. <u>X-inactivation profile reveals extensive variability in X-linked gene expression in females</u>. 17 March 2005. *Nature.* 434(7031):400-4.

2. <u>Ozone Can Affect Heavier People More</u>. Online. 27 November 2007.
<http://www.niehs.nih.gov/news/releases/2007/ozone.cfm>
Reference: W.D. Bennett; M.J. Hazucha; L.J. Folinsbee; P.A. Bromberg; G.E. Kissling; S.J. London. <u>Acute Pulmonary Function Response to Ozone in Young Adults as a Function of Body Mass Index</u>. Inhalation Toxicology, 2007 19 (14): 1147-1154

3. Michael Smith. <u>Fitness Predicts Lower Stroke Risk</u>. Online. 10 December 2007.
<http://www.medpagetoday.com/Cardiology/Strokes/tb/7642>
Reference: P.K. Myint et al "Physical health-related quality of life predicts stroke in the EPIC-Norfolk" *Neurology* 2007; 69: 2243-48.

4. Dr. James Laditka; Dr. Steven N. Blair; Dr. Mei Sui; Dr. James W. Hardin; Dr. Steven P. Hooker; Nancy Chase. <u>JAMA report: Fitness seniors live longer</u>. Online. 4 December 2007.
<http://uscnews.sc.edu/2007/HLTH330-07.html>
Reference: 12/5/07 issue of The Journal of the American

Medical Association.

5. Dr. Donohue. "Older adults who are physically strong have fewer balance problems." St. Louis Post-Dispatch. 2 February 2008.

6. Maura K. Whiteman, PhD; Catherine A. Staropoli, MD; Patricia W. Langenberg, PhD; Robert J. McCarter, ScD; Kristen H. Kjerulff, PhD; Jodi A. Flaws, PhD. Smoking, Body Mass, and Hot Flashes in Midlife Women. *Obstetrics & Gynecology* 2003;101:264-272 © 2003 by The American College of Obstetricians and Gynecologists.

7. American Academy of Neurology. High BMI Tied To Poor Cognitive Function In Middle-Aged Adults. ScienceDaily. 11 October 2006. Online. 19 April 2008. <http://www.sciencedaily.com/¬releases/2006/10/061010023000. htm>

Chapter 2

1. Dr. Donohue. "The risk of illness for an obese person is 50% greater than for a person of normal weight." St. Louis Post-Dispatch. 5 February 2008.

2. The Weight Watchers Research Department. Aging and Metabolism. April 2006. Online. 7 May 2008. <http://www.weightwatchers.com/util/art/index_art.aspx?tabnum =1&art_id=24491&sc=801>

3. Neil Osterweil. Fighting 40s Flab. 5 May 2004. Online. 7 May 2008. <http://www.webmd.com/solutions/sc/lose-weight-for-life/metabolism-rut>

Chapter 4

1. National Center for Health Statistics. Online. 15 May 2008. <http://www.cdc.gov/nchs/data/hus/hus04trend.pdf#069>

Chapter 6

1. 10 Unusual Fad Diets. 13 May 2007. Online. 24 June 2008. <http://www4.vindy.com/content/entertainment/30599262818461 7.php>

2. Kathy Jones. Protein-Rich Meals Trigger Satiety Hormone. 6 September 2006. Online. 18 May 2008.

<http://www.foodconsumer.org/777/8/Protein-Rich_Meals_Trigger_Satiety_Hormone_.shtml>

Chapter 7

1. Nanci Hellmich. "Study suggests eating slowly translates to eating less." <u>USA Today</u>. 15 November 2006. Online. 18 May 2008.
<http://www.usatoday.com/news/health/2006-11-15-slower-eating_x.htm>

2. <u>Increased Fiber Curbs Appetite in Women</u>. 1 November 2002. Online. 21 May 2008.
<http://www.sciencedaily.com/releases/2002/11/021101070442.htm>

3. American Heart Association. <u>How did Americans Get So Heavy?</u> Online. 18 May 2008.
<http://www.americanheart.org/presenter.jhtml?identifier=3040447>

4. Fiona Macrae. <u>Why eating soup could help you lose weight</u>. 2 May 2007. Online. 20 May 2008.
<http://www.dailymail.co.uk/health/article-452198/Why-eating-soup-help-lose-weight.html>

5. <u>Skipping breakfast very bad for health</u>. 26 July 2003. Online. 20 May 2008.
<http://www.medicalnewstoday.com/articles/4004.php>

6. Dr. Maoshing Ni. <u>New Year's Weight Loss: Six Tips</u>. 18 December 2007. Online. 2 June 2008.
<http://health.yahoo.com/experts/drmao/8305/new-years-weight-loss-6-tips/>

7. "Double dipping? 'Seinfeld' was right." <u>USA Today</u>. 2 February 2008. Online. 20 May 2008.
<http://www.usatoday.com/news/health/2008-02-01-double-dipping_N.htm>

8. <u>Concerned Health Experts Investigate Roots of "The Clean Plate Club"</u>. 12 September 2003. Online. 21 May 2008.
<http://www.aicr.org/site/News2?abbr=pr_&page=NewsArticle&id=7526>

9. P. Haines; M. Hama; D. Guilkey. Americans eat more calories on weekends compared to weekdays - Energy Intake. Nutrition Research Newsletter. September 2003. Online. 21 May 2008.

<http://findarticles.com/p/articles/mi_m0887/is_9_22/ai_108879729>

Chapter 8

1. Archives of Internal Medicine, Vol. 165 No. 20. Effects of Physical Activity on Life Expectancy with Cardiovascular Disease. 14 November 2005. Online. 24 May 2008.
<http://archinte.ama-assn.org/cgi/content/abstract/165/20/2355?maxtoshow=&HITS=10&hits=10&RESULTFORMAT=&fulltext=physical+activity&searchid=1&FIRSTINDEX=0&resourcetype=HWCIT>
2. Miranda Hitti. Exercise helps prevent breast cancer. 16 February 2007. Online. 23 May 2008.
<http://www.webmd.com/breast-cancer/news/20070216/exercise-helps-prevent-breast-cancer>
3. Gary Heavin; Carol C. Colman. Reprint edition. 7 December 2004. *Curves: Permanent Results Without Permanent Dieting.*
4. Exercise chops cold risk for older women, study suggests. 26 October 2006. Online. 23 May 2008.
<http://www.cbc.ca/story/health/national/2006/10/26/exercise-colds.html?ref=rss>
5. The Bottom Line on Fitness. 8 December 2003. Online. 24 June 2008.
<http://www.abilitymagazine.com/news_fitness.html>

Chapter 9

1. Archives of Internal Medicine, Vol. 168 No. 2. Association Between Physical Activity in Leisure Time Leukocyte Telemere Length. 28 January 2008. Online. 24 2008.
<http://archinte.ama-assn.org/cgi/content/short/168/2/154>
2. Catherine Keefe. "Spouses who exercise together better chance of sticking to fitness plan." Ridder/Tribune News Service. 29 January 1996. On May 2008.
<http://www.highbeam.com/doc/1G1-17882557.html>
3. "Exercise linked to 'younger' DNA". The Ph Inquirer and The Washington Post. 29 January 200 24 May 2008.

<http://seattletimes.nwsource.com/html/nationworld/2004150728
_exercise29.html>

4. Michael Mosley. <u>Science: Fidget Pants</u>. 25 May 2008.
Online. 25 May 2008.
<http://www.bbc.co.uk/theoneshow/article/2008/01/
mm_fidgetpants.shtml>

5. Malcolm Simmonds. <u>Exercise: Essential for Circulation</u>.
June 2002. Online. 25 May 2008.
<http://www.alternative-healthzine.com/html/0206.html>

6. Julie Deardorff. <u>Why you need green exercise</u>. 5 February
2008. Online. 25 May 2008.
<http://featuresblogs.chicagotribune.com/features_julieshealthclub
/2008/02/the-best-brain.html>

7. Jonathan D. Meeks; Robert T. Herdegen. <u>Music enhances
exercise performance but not physiological recovery following
exercise</u>. 21 June 2002. Online. 25 May 2008.
<http://216.109.125.130/search/cache?ei=UTF-8&p=hampden-
ydney+college+study+exercise&fr=slv1-
be&u=www2.hsc.edu/academics/psychology/staff/herdegen/res
chpapers/aps02exercisebike.doc&w=hampden+sydney+college+
+exercise&d=Xu63FfL9PxHp&icp=1&.intl=us>

enise Gellene. <u>Walk, count, lose weight</u>. 21 November
Online. 25 May 2008.
www.boston.com/news/health/articles/2007/11/21/walk
se_weight/>

arcia. <u>Back pain? Tips to help you cope</u>. 25
7. Online. 26 May 2008.
nonsandiego.com/uniontrib/20070925/news_1c25

avant. "Ask Marilyn." <u>Parade Magazine</u>. 10

e water burn calories? 17 August 2000.
Online. 26 May 2008.
orks.com/question447.htm>

akes you fat. 2 July 2007. Online. 26

news/National/Its-official--stress-
3351105088.html>

Finds Chewing Gum May Help

Reduce Cravings and Control Appetite. 23 October 2007. Online. 26 May 2008.
<http://www.medicalnewstoday.com/articles/86387.php>

Made in the USA
Lexington, KY
02 January 2017